D1296633

L❤VE YOUR GUT

The Experiment, LLC
220 East 23rd Street, Suite 600
New York, NY 10010-4658
theexperimentpublishing.com

Library of Congress Cataloging-in-Publication Data

Names: Rossi, Megan, author.
Title: Love your gut : supercharge your digestive health and transform
   your well-being from the inside out / Megan Rossi.
Description: New York : The Experiment, 2021. | Includes index.
Identifiers: LCCN 2020042330 (print) | LCCN 2020042331 (ebook) | ISBN
   9781615197064 (paperback) | ISBN 9781615197071 (ebook)
Subjects: LCSH: Gastrointestinal system--Diseases--Diet therapy. |
   Digestive organs--Diseases--Diet therapy. | Cooking--Health aspects.
Classification: LCC RC806 .R68 2021 (print) | LCC RC806 (ebook) | DDC
   616.3/3--dc23
LC record available at https://lccn.loc.gov/2020042330
LC ebook record available at https://lccn.loc.gov/2020042331

ISBN 978-1-61519-706-4
Ebook ISBN 978-161519-707-1

Cover and text design by Jack Dunnington
Author photograph by Emma Croman

Manufactured in Turkey

First printing January 2021
10 9 8 7 6 5 4 3 2 1

L♥VE
Y◯UR
GUT

**Supercharge Your Digestive Health
and Transform Your Well-Being
from the Inside Out**

DR. MEGAN ROSSI

THE EXPERIMENT

NEW YORK

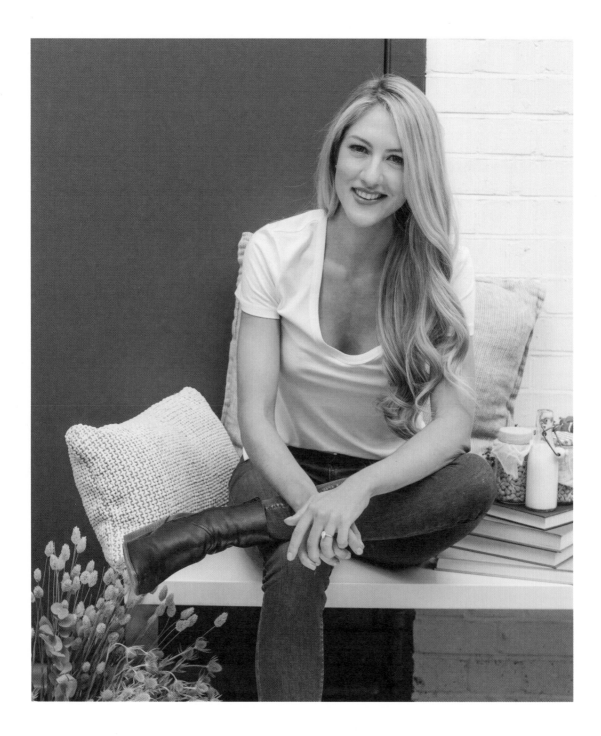

In loving memory of my sister Justine, nephew Boyd, and grandma Ruth—
you inspire me every day. This book is for you.

Contents

Introduction

The Start of Something Beautiful

THE GUT. A simple yet powerful three-letter word and something I have come to think of as beautiful. Yes, I know what you're thinking—it's where poop comes from, for crying out loud! I get it. I used to think the same, but by the time you get to the end of this book, I'm going to have you talking about your gut with a newfound level of admiration and even a dash of excitement. So, let me introduce you. . . .

Say hello to what we nerdy scientists call your gut microbiota (GM). I'm aware it's not the sexiest of terms—so let's go with GM moving forward. This wonderful, complex, and thriving community is made up of the trillions of microbes that call your intestine home. Your GM is incredibly powerful—in fact, this newly appreciated organ is pretty much essential to whatever your health goal is. It's not only capable of thousands of functions, going well beyond what we could achieve on our own, but it has also been linked with successful weight management, improved fitness levels, healthier skin, boosted immunity, and even our happiness.

What really blows my mind is that, unlike our genetic makeup, over which we have no control, we have the ability to shape our GM simply by how we treat it—from getting plenty of fiber and diverse plant goodness to keeping on top of our sleep, stress, and exercise—which means that a big part of our personal health is in our hands. However, as with all landmark scientific discoveries, there are those who will seek to take advantage of people looking for help by twisting the truth and promoting overhyped, sham gut-boosting products. But don't let this detract from the fact that the field of gut health is based on real science and has the potential to have a measurable impact on your health and happiness. In this book, I want to create a safe place to learn about the gut that's all about keeping it real by sticking with the evidence.

The concept of gut health is really nothing new. You see, our GM is just one part of overall gut health. Other major aspects include its role in our immunity (70 percent of immune cells live along the gut), as well as in digestion and the absorption of nutrients, which, if not working right, can lead to an array of nutrition deficiencies and negative health consequences. So, clearly, taking the time to understand and look after our gut is one of the best ways we can invest in our future.

There is a growing and frankly concerning trend toward generic, oversimplified, one-size-fits-all gut-health recommendations. I'm sure you've all heard it before: "Eat more probiotics," "Eat more fermented foods" . . . and on and on. These messages, although I'm sure they're mostly given with good intentions, can actually do more harm than good. An example of this is the contradictory message that everyone should be eating more prebiotics (essentially food for your microbes) if they want good gut health. My research, and research done by others, has clearly demonstrated that for around 15 to 20 percent of the population, particularly those with irritable bowel syndrome (IBS), adding

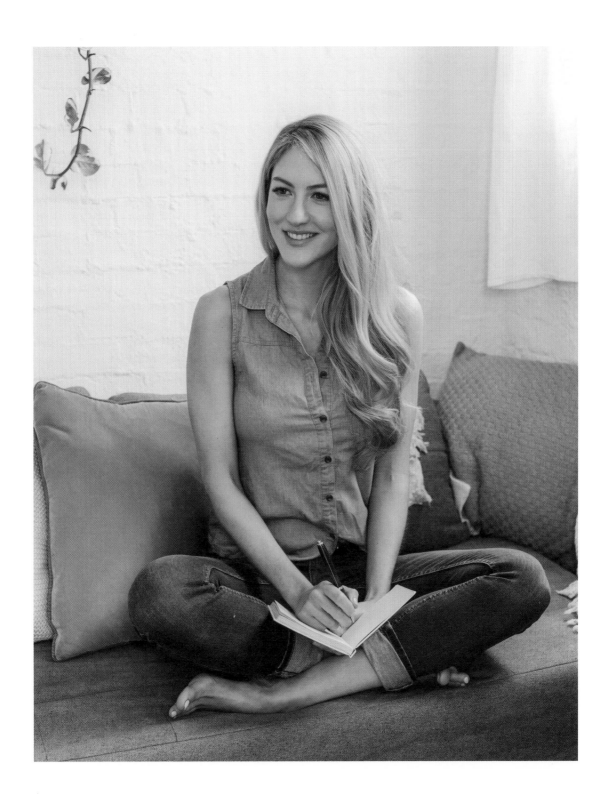

extra prebiotics into your diet can in fact trigger gut symptoms. Yes, of course increasing prebiotics in your diet can be good for you, but it really does depend on where you are on your gut-health journey.

How do you know what's right for you? In this book, we'll go through several assessments (just as I would in my clinic) to help you determine where your gut health is currently at, and then, based on this, we'll explore a range of tools and strategies so that you can formulate your own evidence-based gut-health action plan. All assessments in this book can also be found on my website, theguthealthdoctor.com/book. Record your scores in your Gut-Health Action Plan on page 201.

I do need to prepare you, though: Things are going to get real personal—there's no hiding behind a generic meal plan here. This book is written in a way that I hope not only makes you fall in love with your gut (as I have with mine) but also helps you get the most out of it, whether it's managing existing gut symptoms or maximizing your gut health's impact on other organs, such as your brain. Let's face it: It's the same as most relationships; if you don't give it enough love and attention, things can turn pretty ugly.

My goal in writing this book is to give you a reference guide to your gut—how it works, how to look after it, how to maximize its potential and, most importantly, how to manage it with simple steps when it's not functioning quite right. Using the right balance of science, anecdotes, practical strategies, and tasty fiber-filled recipes packed with plant-based diversity (more on that later!), I will take you on a journey of discovery, leaving you with tangible take-home messages and a step-by-step action plan that will make a meaningful and measurable difference to your everyday life. The book will also equip you with the skills needed to separate the facts from the fiction without getting too "sciencey" on you—promise.

It's time to get excited: Your journey of self-discovery and gut love is about to begin!

Assessment: IS MY GUT HEALTHY?

This has to be the most common question I get asked, and it's one I never give a simple yes or no answer to. There's no single measure we can use to assess our gut health. However, with the right set of tools, you can get a pretty good idea of how healthy your gut is without having to step a foot outside your door. This assessment will give you a little more insight into how this book might benefit you. For each of the ten questions, circle the answer that applies to you.

1. How often are you bothered by gut symptoms (e.g., bloating, reflux, constipation)?

Less than once a month (0 points)	1 to 3 times a month (1 point)	1 to 2 times a week (2 points)	3 or more times per week (3 points)

2. Do you take regular medication or over-the-counter drugs (including the contraceptive pill)?

No (0 points)	Yes (2 points)

3. Do any health conditions run in your family (e.g., diabetes, high blood pressure)?

No	Yes
(0 points)	(2 points)

4. How many different plant-based foods do you eat each week? (Include whole grains, legumes, vegetables, fruits, nuts, and seeds; herbs and spices count as a quarter of a food.)

Fewer than 10	10 to 19	20 to 29	30+
(3 points)	(2 points)	(1 point)	(0 points)

5. In an average week, how would you describe yourself?

Unhappy	Neutral	Happy
(2 points)	(1 point)	(0 points)

6. How often are you unwell (e.g., with colds and flu)?

Fewer than 3 times a year	Once every 2 to 4 months	At least once a month
(0 points)	(1 point)	(2 points)

7. Are you avoiding any foods because of a suspected or diagnosed food intolerance?

No	Yes
(0 points)	(2 points)

8. How many hours of sleep do you get a night on average?

5 hours or fewer	More than 5 hours and fewer than 7 (1 point)	At least 7 hours
(2 points)		(0 points)

9. How often are you negatively impacted by stress?

Less than once a month	1 to 3 times a month	Every week
(0 points)	(1 point)	(2 points)

10. How often do you exercise (for at least 30 minutes) to a level where you'd become short of breath if you tried to sing?

Less often than once a week	1 to 2 times per week	3 or more times a week
(2 points)	(1 point)	(0 points)

Your score : _____

SCORE INTERPRETATION

Great job! For you, it's all about keeping your gut health in top condition. To help you achieve this, keep reading for simple tips on gut health and gut-loving recipes (see page 216).

Let's get to work! Using the practical strategies laid out in this book, we'll get your gut health back on track—it's all about health and happiness from the inside out.

0 points ➡ **20 points**

My Story

I grew up on a farm just outside of Cairns, Australia, where our lifestyle was inherently supportive of good gut health—we played in the dirt and lived on fresh, home-grown produce—yet my first conscious memory of the gut wasn't a happy one. It was during my nutrition and dietetics undergraduate studies, when my grandma, the most caring soul, was diagnosed with bowel cancer. I remember watching helplessly as she bravely battled through chemo and surgery—I hated the gut for doing this to her. Grandma fought as long as she could but lost her battle in 2009, during my final year of college. I still vividly recall sitting in class soon after she'd passed, being taught about the early warning signs of bowel cancer and thinking to myself, *I wonder if talking about our bowels weren't such a socially taboo topic, would my granny have spoken up earlier and still be here today?* The statistics suggested that yes, she would be.

A few years later, those negative emotions surrounding the gut resurfaced. I was working in a hospital as a dietitian and was struck by the sheer number of patients with kidney disease who were complaining of gut issues. I really struggled to get my head around how, while my grandma's disease had been in her actual gut, all these patients with their various kidney diseases also suffered such prominent gut issues. I searched just about every textbook and research paper I could find and still couldn't give my patients a proper answer. But I couldn't let it rest. I was determined to get to the bottom of it, and before I knew it, I found myself signing away my early twenties to answer this very question: Was there a link between the kidneys and the gut?

Fast-forward a few years, and it turns out there is! It's something we now call the gut-kidney axis. But my fascination with the subject didn't stop there. I was fortunate

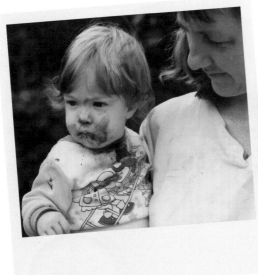

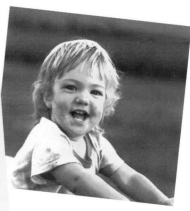

to also work with Olympic athletes and a number of company CEOs, and they got me thinking about the link between the gut and the brain (commonly referred to as the gut-brain axis). I noticed that those who were suffering the greatest levels of stress were the ones suffering the most significant gut issues. It also became clear that, by nourishing the gut and caring for it, people could improve their lives in very real and often surprising ways, and I could help them to do this. This was the turning point in my relationship with the gut—my eyes were finally opened to its power and promise.

So why this book? I went into research to make a difference, but a year into my post-doctoral position at a gut clinic, I became frustrated that, despite the incredible research that was being done, unfounded and potentially dangerous fad nutritional messages were being almost force-fed to the public. I was seeing extremes in my clinic, with some people essentially starving themselves because they'd had (invalid) food-intolerance tests and were scared to eat anything, while others (and I'm talking really intelligent people) were overdosing on herbal supplements in order to "boost" their gut health because they'd read about the gut-brain axis and wanted that extra "edge" at work. Looking after your gut health is not about restrictive diets or taking expensive supplements, yet right before my eyes, I was seeing that the very thing I had come to admire—the gut—was being misrepresented and destroying people's health. It was this injustice that ignited my passion for science communication—to educate and empower people to enjoy good gut health, without the fads. This, along with your endless support on social media, continues to drive my mission to help people find inspiration and take evidence-based steps to a happy, healthy life. But that's quite enough about my story. This book is all about your journey.

So, let's get started!

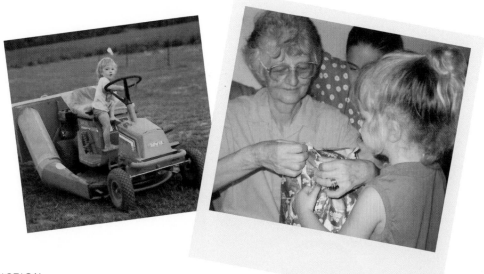

CHAPTER 1

Understanding Your Gut

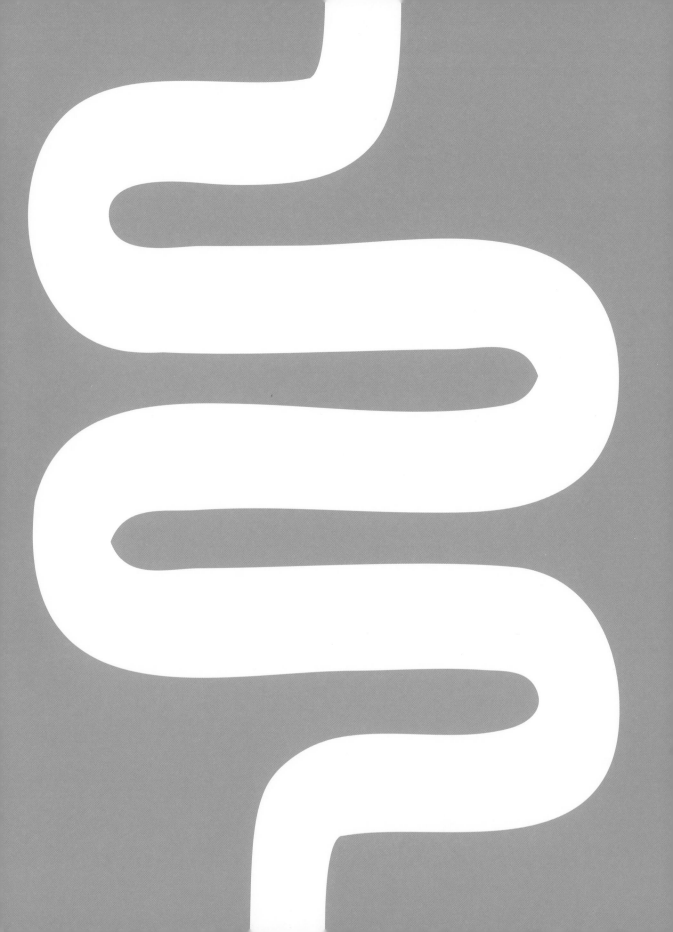

Understanding Your Gut

One of the most important and fundamental things you will ever learn about nutrition is this: what actually happens to food once it enters your mouth.

Why is this knowledge so important? For those who suffer from gut issues, it can help you understand the possible causes. Not only does this help you become a better detective when we come to try and identify any triggers in chapter 5, but having this improved awareness of what goes on inside us can also offer a huge amount of relief. Gut issues aside, by understanding how your body handles food, you're also safeguarding yourself against the many nutrition myths out there, such as the claim that sucrose (aka sugar) is bad for your gut microbes. (Spoiler alert: It's absorbed higher up your intestine, so it doesn't reach the majority of them.)

Despite the hype around our gut microbiota (GM), gut health relates to our entire digestive tract. This means gut health is not just about the microbes. It also includes the digestion of food and the absorption of nutrients, and it maintains most of our immune system. In fact, only a small section of our 30-foot-long (9 m) factory line (aka our digestive tract) contains the bulk of our GM.

Our digestive tract is the barrier between our body and the environment. This means that food doesn't really get into our body until long after we've eaten it—after it has passed through our gut lining's defense barrier and into our bloodstream. If you think about it, this is a huge responsibility for our gut, and it explains why it's equipped with an incredible 70 percent of our body's immune cells.

So, let's take a look at what happens to food as it travels through our body. . . .

In Your Mouth

This is where digestion begins. Food is not only physically broken down in our mouth into smaller bits by our teeth, it's also chemically broken down, thanks to special proteins in our saliva known as enzymes. For example, if you keep a piece of white bread in your mouth for long enough, the enzymes start to break down the complex carbohydrates (starch) and release simple carbohydrates (sugars). As this chemical process happens in your mouth, you will notice that the bread will start to taste sweet—give it a try.

In Your Esophagus

Once you swallow your chewed food, it slides down your food pipe (aka esophagus). To stop the food from going down your windpipe, which is right next to the food pipe, a special trapdoor known as the epiglottis slams shut over your windpipe when you swallow. Have you ever tried to speak and swallow at the same time? It's impossible, without choking, and that's all thanks to our epiglottis.

In Your Stomach

As food travels down your esophagus to your stomach, it needs to pass another circular ring of muscle known as the lower esophageal sphincter. As food moves into each of the next three sections of your digestive tract, it passes through another gateway, or sphincter, at each stage. These sphincters are important, as they keep the different sections separate. Sometimes, however, they don't shut or open properly, which can result in common complaints such as acid reflux and other conditions, which we'll discuss in chapter 4.

You can think of the stomach as a kind of washing machine, because it not only physically churns and throws food around like a washing machine does our clothes, but it also releases detergent-like chemicals. They include:

1. ENZYMES: to break up our food

2. ACID: to kill off pathogens trying to invade our body

3. HORMONES: to trigger the gut muscles to get their act together and start contracting and also let us know when we are full or hungry.

It's in your stomach that your once-solid meal will be transformed to have a more smoothie-like consistency (known as chyme). Once formed, this smoothie mix makes its way from the stomach into the next section of our digestive tract: the small intestine.

In Your Small Intestine

"Small intestine" is bit of a funny name for it, because it's the longest part of our digestive tract, reaching close to 23 feet (7 m) in length when stretched out. If it were laid out flat, it would cover the surface area of nearly half a badminton court! It achieves this impressive surface area with tiny, carpet-like pro jections (villi and microvilli) that exist along its length. These projections are vital for nutrient absorption, that is, the movement of nutrients from our gut into our circulation. In scenarios where these fingerlike projections are flattened or squashed, such as in undiagnosed celiac disease, you are likely to suffer from nutrient deficiencies, partly because your small intestine just doesn't have the surface area needed to absorb all the nutrients from your food. Before the smoothie mix can move into our circulation, it needs to be broken down further, which is where the pancreas comes in. Our pancreas is another organ that feeds into our small intestine. It acts like a busy factory, producing enzymes, which help digest our food, and hormones, which help control how much sugar is in our blood.

To further assist with digestion, yet another detergent-like mix, known as bile acids, is made by our liver and stored in a small pouch known as the gallbladder. Bile is secreted into our small intestine and helps with fat digestion and absorption.

In addition to the enzymes released by our pancreas, the lining of our small intestine also contains enzymes that break down food. For example, lactase, an enzyme that breaks down lactose (a type of sugar found in milk from animals), perches on the lining of your small intestine, waiting to do its job at a moment's notice.

After around two to six hours in your small intestine—depending on what and how much you've eaten, as well as how your gut muscles are working—the unabsorbed bits (including my own personal favorite nutrient, dietary fiber) will move through the next gateway (this one is called the ileocecal valve) and on into the large intestine. As the food passes through this gateway, our large intestine acts a bit like a watchdog, keeping an eye on the things that are passing through. If it starts to notice underdigested food coming through, it pulls the brake on our upper-gut movements. This system is known as the ileal brake, and it's an important feedback system that helps maximize nutrient absorption in the small intestine. One of the side effects of this is decreased appetite, which explains why, when we have diarrhea, we also often lose our appetite.

In Your Large Intestine

The large intestine is responsible for four main things.

1. HYDRATION: Your large intestine reabsorbs fluid and electrolytes. During this process, your gut contents turn from liquid to solid. The longer your poop-to-be is in the large intestine, the more water your body absorbs and therefore the more solid your poop becomes.

2. OUR GM RESIDENTS: Your large intestine houses the trillions of microbes that make up the GM. Although we have microbes scattered throughout our digestive tract, this is where the main bulk of microbes hang out. We'll chat more about this in chapter 2.

3. NUTRIENT ABSORPTION: Most of the nutrient absorption occurs in the small intestine, but the large intestine also plays a pivotal role. This is because our GM helps digest things that are indigestible to human enzymes, such as fiber. In doing so, our microbes produce messenger molecules that are capable of many things, such as messaging our brain to say, "OK, you can stop eating now, thanks, we're full," as well as reducing gut inflammation, and much more.

4. WASTE COMPACTION: The end of our large intestine—the rectum—stores and compacts the waste produced by the body, including the parts of dead red blood cells that make our poop brown. Once our brain gives our rectum the all clear, the accumulated waste is released through our final digestive-tract gateway and out through the muscular opening known as the anus.

Unlike our small intestine, our large intestine plays the slow and steady game. This is why undigested foods take around twelve to thirty hours to move through it, despite the large intestine being around four times shorter than the small intestine.

How the Gut Moves

We've discussed a lot about what happens in each part of the gut, but we haven't yet addressed how food actually moves through it.

Your first thought might be that it's all down to gravity, but remember, the gut is close to 30 feet (9 m) of folded intestines, which means that sometimes food has to move against gravity. To allow for this, our digestive tract is coated with both long and circular muscles, which contract in a symphony of orchestrated patterns to guide food on its extraordinary journey through the gut. This is known as motility.

Several "programmed" movements are responsible for the transportation of food between different parts of the digestive tract, and they differ depending on whether we have eaten or not. One of the two basic types of programmed movements is peristaltic waves, which pump food along the gut; the other is segmentation contractions, which help to mix all the gut contents together, including food and enzymes, like a big pot of warm soup.

Programmed movements may be coordinated into higher-level motility patterns. The best example is the migrating motor complex (MMC), which typically moves from the stomach through the small intestine, essentially sweeping the intestine clean between meals. The MMC is like a street sweeper. It sweeps any leftover bits of waste into the large intestine, as well as any microbes that may have crept up unannounced from our large intestine. Next time you hear your belly rumble, don't stress out; it's likely just your intestinal "housekeeper," aka the MMC, doing its thing. This movement occurs every forty-five minutes to two hours, but only between meals (that is, in the fasted state) and generally when you are sleeping. It's one of the many reasons why sleeping is so important for the gut; we'll touch on this in chapter 7. Dysfunction of the MMC may also play a role in some gut disorders, such as small intestinal bacterial overgrowth (SIBO), which we'll discuss on page 164.

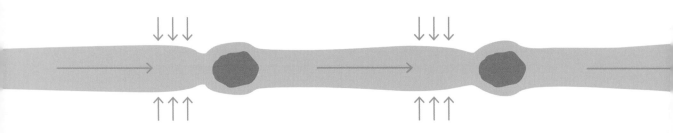

Mass movement is another type of programmed movement, which occurs between six and ten times a day in the large intestine. This is the final "kick," so to speak, propelling your formed poop into your rectum, ready for evacuation. One of the main triggers of this mass movement is eating (known as the gastrocolic reflex: that urge to go that you often feel after eating). It's also worth noting that different foods are thought to have different effects on this type of movement; for instance, fat and carbohydrates are more likely to stimulate this movement than protein. Gentle exercise, such as going for a walk, particularly after a meal, is also known to activate it. Mass movements are put on hold overnight but pick up again sharply when we wake up, which also explains why many people poop in the morning.

So . . . What Makes Your Gut Muscles Contract?

Our gut is really pretty impressive in that, unlike any other organ, it can function independently of our brain. This means that our gut can go about its business, digesting and moving food along, without our brain telling it to do so. This high-level function is all thanks to our gut's impressive network of hundreds of millions of nerves, known as the enteric nervous system. This is why our gut has been dubbed our second brain.

Despite this impressive level of independence, a two-way communication normally occurs between the enteric nervous system and our primary ("big") brain. Much of this communication occurs via our parasympathetic nerves, which is often referred to as the "rest and digest" response, and our sympathetic nerves, which take over when in "fight or flight" response. Typically, when our body feels stressed (because our brain is telling it that we are), the parasympathetic nervous system is regulated downward and so gut function is reduced, because all the blood rushes to our muscles to get them ready to fight (or flee). When we are relaxed, blood goes back into our gut to support digestion. This may explain why some people struggle to poop when they're stressed. Of course, that's not always the case: For some, stress can trigger diarrhea. This is due to overactive or hyperresponsive gut-motility programming, as well as extra fluid being secreted into the gut. The gut-brain link is clearly complex!

Defense System

The gut is the reason we're not all bedridden and defeated by infection every time we eat or step outside. Like all powerhouses, our body has two main lines of defense: the frontline defense of our intestinal wall, which acts as a physical barrier to foreign invaders (like a bouncer at the door outside a club); and the second-line defense of our more sophisticated and dynamic immune system (think security cameras, alarms, and so on).

The wall of our intestine is made up of a barrier of cells (think of a row of doors) that are effectively secured by tight junctions (club bouncers). The intestinal wall serves a dual purpose; like the door and the bouncer who guards it, it allows the passage of the good guys (nutrients) and keeps out the bad guys (pathogens). These tight junctions can become weak, or loose, allowing unwanted nasties to sneak across the intestinal wall. Scientists call this intestinal hyperpermeability, but it's also been referred to as "leaky gut." When talking about a leaky gut, I think it's important to be aware that all our guts become slightly leaky from time to time, without any negative health consequences. We cover this more on page 165, where I talk about whether a leaky gut really is the root of your health problems. (Spoiler alert: No, it's not!) Thankfully, even if a pathogen does make it through the first line, our immune system is primed and waiting to pounce, triggering a cascade of events both within and outside our gut to shut down any nasty invasions.

The immune system is amazingly complex, involving a high-level network of cells, tissues, and organs that work together to fight off invaders. The 70 percent of immune tissue that lies within our gut—our gut-associated lymphoid tissue (GALT)—has a particularly important job, because our digestive tract is the most popular gateway into the body. It's a pretty tough job, really: The team is constantly on patrol, sifting through millions of foreign cells each day (from things we eat and drink, as well as our resident GM), discriminating between the harmless (e.g., proteins in foods and friendly microbes) and potentially dangerous ones (e.g., toxins and pathogenic microbes).

The GALT isn't just important for fighting invaders; it also keeps the rest of our cells and GM in check. This includes performance-assessing old cells that have been subject to extensive wear and tear (and deciding which ones should be made to retire), and good microbes that "act up" and find themselves in the wrong place (that is, crossing the gut barrier).

What happens when things go wrong, when this delicate balance between fighting off the bad guys (immunity) and recognizing the good guys (immune tolerance) is compromised? If the balance tends more toward immunity, conditions such as food allergies (when innocent food proteins are mistakenly tagged as a threat) and autoimmune diseases (where it's the body's own tissues that get tagged) arise. If it tends more toward immune tolerance (often referred to as immunocompromised), as in the case of during certain cancer treatments (e.g., chemotherapy), your body can be more vulnerable to invasion by the bad guys, which may lead to severe infections.

What about your GM? They have a major role in our body's defense system; in fact, without them, our immune system would, frankly, be pretty weak. This is because the microbes train our immune system from birth. This explains the "hygiene hypothesis," which states that being too clean, particularly in infancy, means that you are exposed to fewer microbes, and so your GM diversity (the number of different types of microbes you house) decreases. As a result, the "coaching" of your immune system is also reduced. This is one explanation for why rates of allergy and autoimmune conditions are reaching epidemic levels in the Western world.

Assessment: LISTENING TO YOUR GUT FEELINGS

Have you ever sat down and had a two-way conversation with your gut? You may be surprised by how much you learn from simply taking the time to listen to it.

Although most of us have a sense of when our gut is not functioning quite right, we rarely pinpoint details of the specific symptoms. But doing so can provide invaluable insight and is really worth it. It can not only help you troubleshoot in a more systematic (and therefore helpful) way, but if you do end up needing to see your primary care physician or dietitian, you can provide them with a great source of information, allowing them more time to carry out a thorough assessment in the short time they have to see you. At the start of all my consultations, I get my patients to fill out this questionnaire to help focus our intervention on the areas most important to them.

Start by asking your gut whether any of the symptoms listed below have caused it any hassle over the past seven days. If the answer is no, you can move on to the Checking In with Your Poop assessment on page 24. If the answer is yes, think about (1) how many times (frequency) and (2) the intensity (severity) of the incidents. Remember, there is no right or wrong answer; it's completely your own perception.

An example of how to complete the questionnaire: If you get abdominal pain twice a week and it's of moderate intensity, complete the form like this:

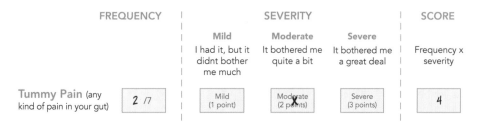

FREQUENCY	SEVERITY			SCORE
	Mild I had it, but it didnt bother me much	**Moderate** It bothered me quite a bit	**Severe** It bothered me a great deal	Frequency x severity
Tummy Pain (any kind of pain in your gut) 2 /7	Mild (1 point)	Moder**X**ate (2 points)	Severe (3 points)	4

Scoring: Multiply the frequency by the severity; e.g., 2 × 2 = 4

	FREQUENCY	SEVERITY			SCORE
		Mild I had it, but it didnt bother me much	**Moderate** It bothered me quite a bit	**Severe** It bothered me a great deal	Frequency x severity
Tummy Pain (any kind of pain in your gut)	/7	Mild (1 point)	Moderate (2 points)	Severe (3 points)	
Heartburn (burning/discomfort behind your breastbone)	/7	Mild (1 point)	Moderate (2 points)	Severe (3 points)	
Acid reflux/acid regurgitation (taste of sour fluid in your mouth)	/7	Mild (1 point)	Moderate (2 points)	Severe (3 points)	
Nausea (feeling sick, with or without vomiting)	/7	Mild (1 point)	Moderate (2 points)	Severe (3 points)	
Belly gurgling/rumbling (vibrations or noise in your gut that cause you discomfort)	/7	Mild (1 point)(	Moderate 2 points)	Severe (3 points)	
Belly bloating (feeling of swelling of your gut; not to be confused with normal bloating after a large meal)	/7	Mild (1 point)	Moderate (2 points)	Severe (3 points)	
Belly distension (physical protrusion of your gut)	/7	Mild (1 point)	Moderate (2 points)	Severe (3 points)	
Belching/burping (bringing up gas through your mouth)	/7	Mild (1 point)	Moderate (2 points)	Severe (3 points)	
Excess flatulence (release of gas from your back end more than twenty times per day)	/7	Mild (1 point)	Moderate (2 points)	Severe (3 points)	
Constipation (infrequent, lumpy, or dry poops)	/7	Mild (1 point)	Moderate (2 points)	Severe (3 points)	
Diarrhea (very frequent, mushy, or watery poops)	/7	Mild (1 point)	Moderate (2 points)	Severe (3 points)	
Urgency (urgent need to poop)	/7	Mild (1 point)	Moderate (2 points)	Severe (3 points)	
Incomplete evacuation (inability to pass all poop)	/7	Mild (1 point)	Moderate (2 points)	Severe (3 points)	
Tiredness (feeling tired despite regularly getting 7 to 9 hours of sleep)	/7	Mild (1 point)	Moderate (2 points)	Severe (3 points)	

Scoring: Add together the individual scores of all your symptoms. Example: If you have abdominal pain (score 6), bloating (score 4), and diarrhea (score 7) your total score would be: 6 + 4 + 7 = 17.

Adapted from Digestive Diseases and Sciences[1]

TOTAL SCORE

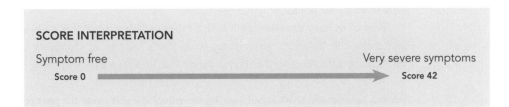

SCORE INTERPRETATION

Symptom free   Very severe symptoms
    Score 0 ————————————————————————▶   Score 42

It's always best to be on the safe side, so if your gut symptoms are accompanied by any of the "Alarm Features" described on page 89, visit your doctor.

How did your conversation with your gut go? Did you learn anything new? Sometimes, we don't realize how much of an impact our gut can have until we take a moment to just sit and listen to it. As a quick side note, it is worth remembering that you can be too conscious of your gut, which can lead to an unhealthy relationship. Yep, it's possible to be too "into" your gut. As with any relationship, you don't want to be neglectful, but then again, you don't want to be overly obsessive either. If you scored on three or more symptoms, it might be worth completing the Gut-Brain Assessment in chapter 4 (see page 89).

You may be wondering how your score compares to others. What is considered "normal" is really quite arbitrary, although research does suggest that as many as 30 percent of us will be bothered by gut symptoms at some stage, so you're not alone! No matter your score, I'm a firm believer that absolutely no one should have to live with uncomfortable gut symptoms. The good news is that there are many simple yet effective strategies to help combat each of these symptoms. Of course, having realistic expectations at the outset is important. Improvements can take over a month to properly manifest themselves, and sometimes we need to accept that these first-line strategies alone aren't enough—at least, initially—but we'll discuss that more in chapter 4.

If you experience tummy pain at least one day a week, you may like to jump to chapter 6 to see if you meet the criteria for irritable bowel syndrome (IBS). If not, let's continue on to the Checking In with Your Poop assessment.

Assessment: CHECKING IN WITH YOUR POOP

We're not taught to consider it so but, believe me, your poop is one of the most underutilized tools to uncover what's going on inside you. It can also let you know when it might be time to visit your doctor.

Most of us have experienced a bout of diarrhea, or a poop that's a bit of a funky color, and that's OK. But if it's an ongoing issue that's happening alongside other symptoms, that's when it deserves further investigation. So, let's take a look at the five steps.

For this assessment, think about your typical pooping habits over the past month.

Step 1: Pooping frequency

On average, how often do you poop?

Less than once per week ☐
1 to 2 times per week ☐
3 to 6 times per week ☐
Once per day ☐
2 to 3 times per day ☐
4 to 6 times per day ☐
More than 6 times per day ☐

If you're regularly pooping more than 3 times a day, it's worth checking in with your doctor.

There are many different factors that affect how frequently we poop, including our diet. And there's actually no such thing as an optimal number, because we're all unique. However, pooping anywhere between three times a week and three times a day is considered "normal."

If you're outside the normal, don't worry. You're not alone: Around 14 percent of adults are thought to have constipation (pooping less than three times per week) and 2 percent have diarrhea (pooping more than three times per day), but it's not something you should have to just put up with. In chapter 4, we'll discuss a range of diet and lifestyle strategies that can help.

Step 2: Time of the day

On average, when do you usually poop?

In the morning ☐
In the afternoon ☐
In the evening ☐
In the middle of the night ☐

If you're waking up at night to poop, it's worth a visit to your doctor.

While most people will poop in the morning, because our gut movements are more active, there's really no right or wrong time to do it. When you have to go, you should go. Holding it in can trigger some undesirable tummy symptoms and, in the long term, can wreak havoc on your digestive system. I do, of course, appreciate that pooping in public places or at a friend's house isn't always the most comfortable thing to do. To help combat those fears, I've developed a special Poop-Pourri recipe that will mask even the strongest of smells (see page 96).

Step 3: Poop consistency

Too few of us check in with the consistency of our poop on a regular basis. This is not to say that you need to be assigning a number to every single poop, but having a general idea of where yours sits on the Bristol Stool Form Scale is more valuable than you may think.

The Bristol Stool Scale

Type 1		Separate hard lumps, like nuts (hard to pass)
Type 2		Sausage-shaped, but lumpy
Type 3		Sausage-shaped, but with cracks on the surface
Type 4		Like a sausage or snake; smooth and soft
Type 5		Soft blobs with clear-cut edges (passed easily)
Type 6		Fluffy pieces with ragged edges; a mushy stool
Type 7		Watery; no solid pieces

Adapted from Scandinavian Journal of Gastroenterology[2]

Are you struggling to pick your "type," because it changes all the time? Rest assured, you're not alone. Around 60 percent of people have different types of poops regularly, meaning it's normal to select a few different types.

If your poop resembles rabbit droppings (type 1), you may want to check out page 90, on managing constipation. If it's on the opposite end of the pooping spectrum (type 6 or 7) and you suffer from other symptoms, such as urgency, head on over to page 100, on diarrhea.

Step 4: Pooping color panel

It's time to talk about color. From time to time, you may have an odd-looking poop but not have any other symptoms. This can happen to anyone and may reflect what you've eaten, like if you've been a bit heavy-handed with beets or kale (which both contain strong color pigments that are difficult to digest). If your poop is consistently strange in color and you also have other symptoms frequently, then it's worth mentioning to your doctor, who can use this as a clue in their assessment.

COLOR	POSSIBLE MEANINGS
Brown	Varying shades of brown are normal. Poop is naturally brown because it contains a chemical called stercobilin, which is a waste product of old red blood cells.
Black	This can be because of excess iron supplements, or it may indicate bleeding in your upper gut. If you're not on any supplements, visit your doctor as soon as possible.
Yellow	This may indicate that your liver isn't happy and, as a result, is not producing enough bile (remember: bile helps to digest fat). It's worth going to see your doctor.
Red	There are many things that can make your poop reddish. It might be due to the natural red pigments in foods such as beets. If you haven't eaten any red foods, it could be blood from the lower part of your intestine. Red blood in the stool can be caused by several things, including hemorrhoids, or it may be an indication of something more sinister, such as inflammatory bowel disease or colon polyps. If it's not food-related, see your doctor as soon as possible.
White/ grey	This means that your poop doesn't contain the brown pigment stercobilin and could suggest that something is wrong with your bile duct. It's worth booking an appointment with your doctor.
Green	Like reddish poop, green shades may be related to your diet, particularly if you're eating a load of dark greens like spinach. It may also be because of a gut infection or antibiotics. If it's not food-related, consult your doctor.

Step 5: Poop size

What about the amount of poop? Don't worry, I'm not going to get you to weigh it out. But this information can be very useful. Larger poops have been linked to a lower risk of colon cancer (with the exception of diarrhea, which is heavy because it's mostly water).

On average, what size are your poops?

Small: Less than 2 ounces/50 g (the equivalent of less than one egg)   ☐
Medium: 2 to 3.5 ounces/50 to 100 g (1 to 2 eggs)   ☐
Large: More than 3.5 ounces/100 g (more than 2 eggs)   ☐

Want to decrease your risk of colon cancer? Dietary fiber is one of the best ways to boost your poop weight. We'll chat more about this in chapter 3.

Remember to record your scores in your Gut-Health Action Plan on page 210.

CHAPTER 2

Your Inner Universe of Microbes

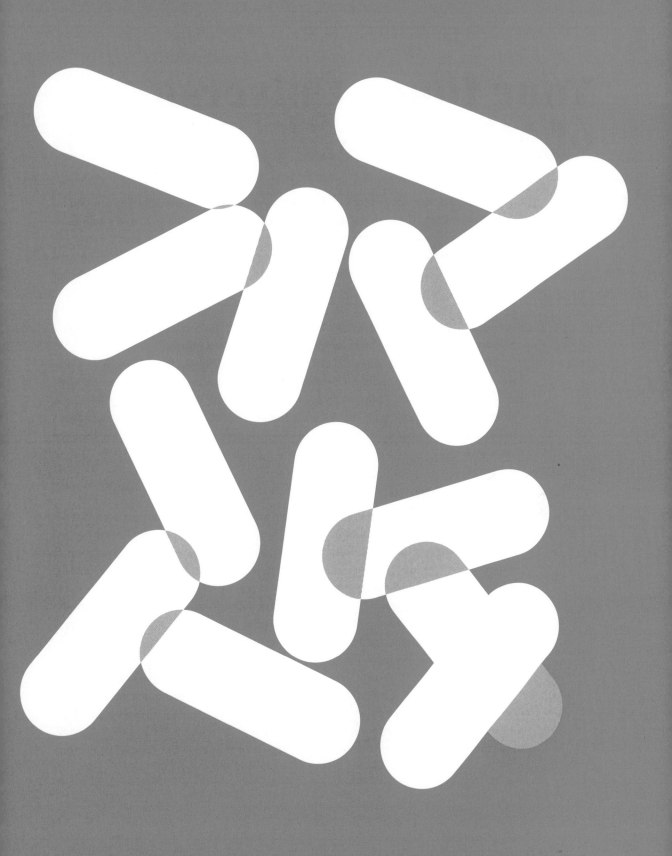

Your Inner Universe of Microbes

Microbes have been around for billions of years, while humans have only been around for less than a million. They can multiply in minutes and survive and thrive in every habitat on Earth, from volcanic explosions to glaciers; they've killed more people than all wars and human accidents combined (not a stat to be proud of, but relevant nonetheless). Perhaps most humbling of all, without microbes, we couldn't survive—but, without us, microbes would do just fine.

Admittedly, this does paint our relationship as a little one-sided, but I can promise you, deep down, your microbes want to see you thrive. As long as you show them some love and appreciation, like all close friends, they'll have your back.

When I talk about microbes, I'm not just talking about our gut microbiota (GM), which we will cover in detail shortly. Our body is in fact like a mini ecosystem of different microbial communities. They live in us—in our lungs, our nose, our urinary tract, and so on—and they also live on us, like a second skin. To microbes, our armpits are like a tropical forest, our backs like a wide open field. Distinct microbe communities populate each area.

Skin Microbiota

We each have billions of microbes living on our skin. We also emit our own distinct cloud of microbes wherever we go, and this is unique, like a fingerprint. This microbial fingerprint, which can't be hidden from others simply by wearing gloves, has grabbed the attention of criminologists as an exciting new forensic tool to hunt down criminals. Perhaps not surprisingly, our skin microbiota also plays a role in common skin conditions like acne, eczema, and certain skin cancers. But before we go getting our hopes up, the ways in which we can manipulate our skin microbes to help prevent and manage those skin conditions are still poorly understood. In terms of preventing eczema in infants, there is supportive evidence that taking probiotics during pregnancy may reduce your baby's risk by up to 50 percent; however, for treating eczema and acne, studies indicate that probiotics don't seem to help. Instead, what's more promising are topical probiotics, where bacteria are directly placed on the skin. But it's still early, so I'd be a little skeptical for now if you come across companies selling "probiotic" skincare. Regarding skin cancers, recent studies in mice have suggested that a specific species of bacteria

(*Staphylococcus epidermidis*) is able to produce a chemical that protects mice against developing skin cancer. Although this finding has yet to be replicated in humans, it suggests that specific skin microbiota may indeed play an important role in protecting against skin cancer. I'm hopeful that in the near future there will be evidence-based products for skincare in humans. But in the meantime, it's best to safeguard yourself by looking into the human research that has been done (not test-tube or animal studies) before handing over your hard-earned cash.

Oral Microbiota

There's also a community of microbes that claim residence in our mouth. These bacteria are notorious for causing bad breath and dental issues, but rest assured that this is the doing of only a select few troublemakers; the vast majority of microbes work to support a healthy mouth environment. They not only act as the bodyguard to our GM but also play several other roles in maintaining our general health. This includes metabolizing specific nutrients, such as nitrates from plants like beets, which can help manage high blood pressure and support heart health.

So how do we look after these guys? Maintaining our oral hygiene, by brushing our teeth properly and regularly and not overdoing it on added sugars—think fizzy drinks and sweets—is a good place to start. One study did report that, with each "intimate" kiss, we transfer an average of 80 million bacteria.[3] This suggests that our partner's diet could also have an impact on our microbes. One of my patients, Claire, was adamant that it was only after her partner started to improve his diet, too, that she started to see results on the scales. Sounds too good to be true? With my scientific hat on, it's more likely that Claire's success was the result of the increased support from her partner and the fewer temptations she was exposed to at home rather than the change in her partner's oral microbes. But that said, the fact that our oral microbiota has been linked to weight gain does pose an interesting thought—and, if nothing else, it may encourage your partner to add a few extra portions of plants into their diet.

For Those of You Who Haven't Yet Met, Say Hello to Your GM

On the face of it, our gut microbes appear quite simple, really, just living their single-celled existence. But it's all just an act. They are, in fact, incredibly smart, which is why you'll find them not randomly scattered but instead strategically located along the gut with other like-minded microbes, forming complex and distinct ecosystems adapted to their environment. There are four key concepts about our GM that are worth knowing.

1. THE BASICS: NOT JUST BACTERIA

When I talk about the GM, I'm not just referring to bacteria but also to other types of microbes, such as fungi and viruses, that live in our gut, too. The fungi is known as our mycobiota, and the virus component is the virome. Although they also play a role in health and disease, our understanding of their function is still at a very early stage. What's even more striking is that some parasites (yes, they live in the gut, too) are said to be more common in healthy people. Those with gut issues such as irritable bowel syndrome (IBS) and inflammatory bowel disease (IBD) have been shown to have fewer, suggesting that some parasites may indeed play a protective role.

2. THE BASICS: THE GOAL IS DIVERSITY

Generally speaking, a higher level of GM diversity is associated with better overall health. The more diverse your GM, the greater the breadth of skills your GM "team" possesses. So just like any soccer team, the most successful isn't the one with all superstar strikers but the one with a range of skills to provide balance. Having a more diverse GM also increases our resilience to infection. It's similar to a thriving garden: If you have all the same plants and a certain disease comes along, it could wipe out your entire garden. But if you have a diverse range of plants, it's very unlikely that one disease has the right array of "weapons" to wipe them all out—some will naturally be resistant. The same goes for your GM. How do you encourage this GM diversity? This is where that all-important fiber- and plant-based diversity comes in (alongside your lifestyle), which we'll look at more in chapter 3.

3. THE BASICS: NO SINGLE IDEAL GM

No two people have the same GM—not even identical twins! When people talk about the GM, they often use the terms *microbiota* and *microbiome* interchangeably. But there's a crucial difference. *Microbiota* refers to the actual community of microbial cells (e.g., bacteria). It's all the genes within these cells that determine what they're capable of doing and how they interact with human cells, and this is what we call the *microbiome*. Different microbiota (groups of microbes) can share similar microbiomes (sets of genes). This leads us to the incredible and fascinating fact that different microbes can perform similar tasks; for example, there are many different bacteria that can produce B vitamins. Another *m* term I feel it's appropriate to bring in at this point is the microbial *metabolome*. This is just a fancy science term to describe the tangible output of what the microbes produce (for example, vitamins and other chemicals). The metabolome is the key to understanding what the microbiota are actually doing. With that in mind, while there's no ideal microbiota, there is a health-associated microbiota for every person, an optimal GM that's just right for you. If you look after your GM with plenty of plant-based foods, by practicing mindfulness and sleeping well, among other strategies we'll discuss, chances are you'll cultivate your own optimal GM.

4. THE BASICS: GOOD VERSUS BAD

Often, microbes are referred to as good or bad. But just like most people, the behavior of any one microbe can be good or bad depending on the environment it finds itself in. Think about yourself: If you've had a poor night's sleep or are so hungry you've reached a state of "hanger" (hunger expressed as anger), then, despite being a genuinely good person, you might get a little grumpy. It turns out our microbes are just like us. For example, *Clostridioides difficile (C. diff)* infection claims thousands of lives in Western countries each year, yet around 3 percent of healthy adults (and 66 percent of babies) have *C. diff* living in their gut. It's only when *C. diff* "acts out" and overgrows, typically in people with weak immunity, that it starts to produce toxins triggering diarrhea and, in severe cases, fever, gut inflammation, and nausea.

What Can It Do for Me?

Now that we have the more formal introductions out of the way, it's time to get down to business and discuss what our GM is actually doing for us. On a day-to-day basis, what are we getting from these guys? To answer this, I have put together a snapshot of the GM's basic skill set. You can think of it as your GM's résumé. When reviewing this, it's worth remembering that résumés are based on your track record, so to speak. This means that there's no guarantee your GM will continue achieving at such a high level going forward if things—your lifestyle, for example—aren't supportive. Of course, if you, as a kind and motivating boss, continue to create a nice "working" environment, there's a strong chance your GM will continue its high-level output. But if the GM is overworked and underpaid, its productivity is likely to take a nosedive.

Our GM and Response to Medication

Ever wondered why your response to a medication may be different from other people's? Although genetics play a key role (between 20 percent and 95 percent, depending on the medication), so does our GM. In fact, different microbes can do different things to medications, including activating or deactivating them, and even converting some into harmful waste products. The latter mechanism is thought to explain, at least in part, why only a subset of people experience severe diarrhea following common colon-cancer chemotherapies, or gut-lining damage after taking anti-inflammatory drugs such as ibuprofen. Our GM may also explain the variable response to certain types of cancer therapies. Indeed, one study found that a more diverse GM was linked to better response to an immune-system therapy in melanoma patients.

If you take regular medication, you may be wondering which microbes you need to improve your success rates and therefore what diet you should be following. Those are the ultimate questions, and ones that hundreds of researchers around the world, including my research group, are working to answer. In the meantime, nurturing your GM with the strategies outlined in the pages to come is the best place to start.

Gut Microbiota's Résumé

- *Can make vitamins (e.g., vitamin K and B vitamins), amino acids (protein building blocks), hormones (e.g., noradrenaline), chemical messengers (e.g., serotonin), and many others.*
- *Trains our immune system.*
- *Produces important molecules that strengthen the gut barrier and may help balance blood sugar, lower blood fats, regulate appetite, facilitate communication with the brain, and ultimately help prevent against many diseases.*
- *Communicates with our other vital organs, including our brain, liver, and heart.*
- *Prevents invasion from bad microbes.*
- *Enjoys eating fiber and antioxidants from a wide variety of plants.*
- *Metabolizes drugs and deactivates toxins.*
- *Influences gut movement and function.*

Assessment: HOW DIVERSE IS YOUR GM?

There are many factors known to affect your GM. Some of them we can change, or at least influence, such as diet (a modifiable factor), and others we can't, such as our age (an unmodifiable factor). The empowering thing about our GM is that so much of it is modifiable—in fact, it turns out that our environment has more of an effect on our GM than our genetics. Targeting our diet is one of the most effective ways we can boost our GM diversity. Most of the research has found that people with high-fiber diets, from a wide range of plant-based foods, have greater GM diversity. So let's begin by looking at how much fiber, plant-based diversity, and additional GM-loving foods you're getting.

This is my version of the validated fiber questionnaire developed by my Australian colleagues Marina Reeves, Elisabeth Winkler, and Elizabeth Eakin.[4] For each question, circle the answer that applies to you, thinking about the past month:

1) How many portions of vegetables did you typically eat each day?
   (1 portion = ½ cup/125 g cooked vegetables or 1 cup of raw vegetables/salad)

0 portions	1 to 2 portions	3 to 4 portions	5 to 6 portions	7+ portions
(0 points)	(1 point)	(2 points)	(3 points)	(4 points)

2) How many portions of fruit did you typically eat each day?
   (1 portion = 1 medium piece, 2 small pieces, 1 cup diced, or 1 ounce/30 g dried)

0 portions	1 portion	2 portions	3 portions	4+ portions
(0 points)	(1 point)	(2 points)	(3 points)	(4 points)

3) How many portions of nuts or seeds did you typically eat each week?
(1 portion = 1 ounce/30 g nuts, e.g., 23 almonds or 1 tablespoon of seeds)

0 portions	1 to 3 portions	4 to 6 portions	7+ portions
(0 points)	(1 point)	(2 points)	(3 points)

4) How often did you eat legumes such as canned beans, lentils, chickpeas, split peas, and dried beans each week?

Never	Less than 1 day	1 to 2 days	3 to 5 days	6 to 7 days
(0 points)	(1 point)	(2 points)	(3 points)	(4 points)

5) How often did you eat a high-fiber breakfast cereal (e.g., bran, oats) each week?

Never	Less than 1 day	1 to 2 days	3 to 5 days	6 to 7 days
(0 points)	(1 point)	(2 points)	(3 points)	(4 points)

6) How often did you choose whole-grain pasta and brown/wild rice instead of white pasta and white rice?

Never	Rarely	Sometimes	Mostly	Always
(0 points)	(1 point)	(2 points)	(3 points)	(4 points)

7) How often did you choose whole-grain bread/crackers/wraps instead of white varieties?

Never	Rarely	Sometimes	Mostly	Always
(0 points)	(1 point)	(2 points)	(3 points)	(4 points)

8) How often did you eat other whole grains (not included in the above; e.g., quinoa, buckwheat, freekeh) each week?

Never	Less than 1 day	1 to 2 days	3 to 5 days	6 to 7 days
(0 points)	(1 point)	(2 points)	(3 points)	(4 points)

Your fiber score: _____

SCORE INTERPRETATION

Very low fiber intake   Very high fiber intake

0 points ————————————————————▶ 31 points

Although fiber has a big impact on our GM's happiness, there are several other dietary components known to impact your GM. Let's take a look at some of these next.

Again, think about the past month:

1) How many different types of plant-based foods did you typically eat each week?
(See page 81 to help you add them all up. Your answer to this question scores triple points, because plant-based foods are thought to have a big impact on GM diversity.)

Fewer than 10	10 to 19	20 to 29	30+
(0 points)	(3 point)	(6 points)	(9 points)

2) Which were you more likely to drink? *(If you don't drink any of these, skip this question.)*

Soft drink	Coffee, tea, or red wine
(-1 point)	(1 point)

3) How many of the top polyphenol (a group of beneficial plant chemicals) foods did you typically eat each week? *(See page 67 for the list of foods, not including herbs and spices.)*

Less than 5	5 to 9	10 to 14	15 to 19	20+
(0 points)	(1 point)	(2 points)	(3 points)	(4 points)

4) How many of the high-polyphenol herbs and spices (see page 67) did you typically eat each week?

Less than 5	5 to 9	10+
(0 points)	(1 point)	(2 points)

5) Did you eat at least one portion of oily fish or three servings of vegetarian sources of omega-3s (such as walnuts, linseeds, chia seeds, or tofu) per week? *(1 portion = 5 ounces/140 g fish, 1 ounce/30 g walnuts, or 1 tablespoon seeds)*

No	Some weeks	Every week
(0 points)	(1 point)	(2 points)

6) How often did you eat fermented food containing live microbes (such as plain probiotic yogurt, kefir, kombucha, or sauerkraut) per week? See page 64 for a list.

Never	Less than 1 day	1 to 2 days	3 to 5 days	6 to 7 days
(0 points)	(1 point)	(2 points)	(3 points)	(4 points)

Your diversity score : _____

Diet-derived GM score (fiber score + diversity score) : _____

SCORE INTERPRETATION

Low diet-derived GM diversity   High diet-derived GM diversity

0 points ➞ **53 points**

How did you do? Keep in mind that this is a very general indicator of the potential GM diversity resulting from your diet, because there are so many factors likely to be at play. We will look at this in more depth in chapter 3.

This brings me to a very important point. Despite the desire to attain high scores, I recognize this isn't always possible for people with gut symptoms. If that's you nodding along right now, put your mind at rest: We'll get you there. The first step is to get those symptoms under control (chapters 4 and 6), and then we'll work on boosting your score.

Central to Health and Well-Being

It's easy to understand how our GM can affect the rest of our gut health, given its close proximity. But it's a little harder to visualize how it could possibly affect other organs that are further afield, like our brain. Thankfully, this concept isn't one we simply need to leave to faith (I am a scientist, after all), as there is mounting scientific evidence that demonstrates just how our GM and our other organs interact with each other.

In the past few years we've come to understand, at least in part, three of the communication styles that our GM tends to use:

1. THE IMMUNE SYSTEM (think: house alarm)

2. THE NERVOUS SYSTEM (think: mobile phone)

3. THE CIRCULATION—that is, the blood and lymphatic system (think: postal service)

Our GM makes full use of each of these, depending on the type of message it wants to send and how quickly it wants to send it. For example, if it's something urgent, like a viral invasion, then it's more likely to pick up the mobile or trigger the alarm to alert the rest of the body rather than relying on "snail mail." However, if it's something slow and gradual, such as a chronic disease, then the GM is fine to send packages via the postal service. To date, specific GM patterns (often called dysbiosis) have been linked with over seventy different conditions. But research is still only in its early stages, meaning we still don't know whether the altered GM contributes to disease (GM is the driver, disease is the passenger) or whether it's the other way around.

Despite this, after over ten years working as a clinician, I'm convinced that everyone can benefit from looking after their GM, whether it directly or indirectly affects a specific condition or not. So, even if you're suffering from a condition where the evidence is still limited in terms of the role of the GM, why not try some of the simple, cost-effective diet strategies in chapter 3 (alongside any necessary medical treatment, of course)? It's best to try out the diet strategies for a four-week period and then assess whether you notice an improvement. What do you have to lose?

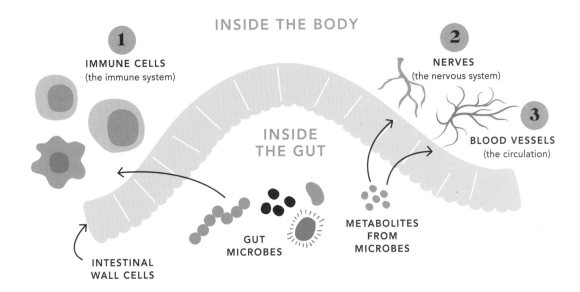

INSIDE THE BODY

1
IMMUNE CELLS
(the immune system)

2
NERVES
(the nervous system)

3
BLOOD VESSELS
(the circulation)

INSIDE
THE GUT

GUT
MICROBES

METABOLITES
FROM
MICROBES

INTESTINAL
WALL CELLS

Gut-Brain Axis

The constant, two-way communication that occurs between our gut and our brain is referred to as the gut-brain axis. The latest evidence suggests that tapping into our gut-brain axis could play a pivotal role in our mental health. With one in four of us predicted to experience a mental health event this year alone, our gut health really is something more of us should be taking into consideration.

Although the science behind the gut-brain axis (particularly how our GM is involved) is relatively new, the "gut feeling" phenomenon is something we've all experienced. In fact, long before science connected the two, we were using gut functions to describe our feelings and emotions: "I've got butterflies in my stomach"; "You don't have the guts for it"; "I can't stomach that behavior" . . . clearly our ancestors were onto something.

Our understanding of the connection between our brain and our GM is still in the early stages, but there's some promising evidence building. Trials have shown not only that our GM is implicated in our mental health but that, by modifying our GM with the simple diet strategies discussed in chapter 3 and the recipes in chapter 9, we can help manage mental health conditions, such as depression (alongside medication and therapy, as needed). What's more, by nourishing our GM with both the diet and non-diet strategies discussed in the chapters to come, we may even be able to prevent some cases of depression and anxiety.

In my practice, I have witnessed the powerful role that diet can play in the management of some people's mental health, including that of twenty-four-year-old Paul. When Paul first walked into my room at the clinic, his shoulders were hunched, his head down, his voice soft, and his words mumbled; it was clear he was going through a tough time. As Paul and I got talking, he opened up about his history of depression, which first started after he moved away for college several years prior. He described himself as having been very sociable before that—he'd been captain of the football team and dated his high school sweetheart—but by the age of twenty-two, he explained, "I'd lost all interest in life." He'd stopped playing sports, broken up with his girlfriend, and distanced himself from his close friends. He saw his family doctor three times over the summer and was prescribed an antidepressant. Although initially hesitant, Paul decided to give the antidepressant a try as he headed back to school. Over the following three months he noticed some improvement in his mood, although he still found himself avoiding social events. As fate would have it, Paul just so happened to be in the waiting room of his college doctor when he stumbled upon an article that I'd written describing one of my favorite clinical trials: the SMILES trial.[5] The article really resonated with Paul, who moments later found himself explaining to his doctor that, although he had come in with a plan to consider increasing his dose of antidepressants, he had just read a convincing article supporting the role of diet and wanted to hold off until he'd had time to look into this further. With his doctor's approval, two weeks later, Paul was sitting in front of me with a rather novel request; he wanted to follow the study I'd written about in that article. So that's exactly what we did. Paul filled out the assessment questionnaires from the study, and I counseled him on the Mediterranean diet, just as the dietitian had done with the trial participants. The diet was high in whole grains, vegetables, fruit, nuts, seeds, legumes, and extra virgin olive oil, and contained nearly three times the dietary fiber most of us eat (as we'll discuss in chapter 3). I reviewed Paul six times over the following twelve weeks, as they had in the study.

I'm not going to paint a false picture and say it was easy. It certainly wasn't. Paul was going from a heavily fast-food-based diet to eating homemade, mostly plant-based meals. At each phone review, Paul talked me through the tough days when he'd end up paying a visit to those devilishly tempting golden arches, and together we troubleshoot (which included using some quick and easy recipes) and moved forward. Now, I'm a big believer in diet, but when Paul walked back into clinic twelve weeks later, sporting the biggest smile, from ear to ear, with the color back in his face and a strong posture, even I was impressed. His first words—"Megan, life is good"—pretty much summed it up. I received an email from him nine months later, where he shared his mom's gratitude with me and his family doctor's decision to lower his antidepressant dose with the goal of stopping them altogether. And for the romantics out there, Paul added that he'd also rekindled his relationship with his high school sweetheart.

Assessment: HOW HAPPY ARE YOU?

This is such an important question, but one that too few of us ask ourselves. So, let's take a look at your current happiness levels.

When completing this assessment, it's best not to take too long thinking about each question. The first answer that comes into your head is probably the right one for you. If you find some of the questions difficult, give the answer that is true for you most of the time.

This questionnaire is a shortened version of the famous Oxford Happiness Questionnaire developed by Peter Hills and Michael Argyle.[6] This is a great questionnaire to repeat after a few months of nurturing your gut using the strategies outlined in the book.

Some of the questions are phrased negatively, others positively, so you'll need to read through each one carefully and really think about each question. Circle one number per question.

	Strongly disagree	Moderately disagree	Slightly disagree	Slightly agree	Moderately agree	Strongly agree
1) I don't feel particularly pleased with the way I am.	6	5	4	3	2	1
2) I feel that life is very rewarding.	1	2	3	4	5	6
3) I am well satisfied about everything in my life.	1	2	3	4	5	6
4) I don't think I look attractive.	6	5	4	3	2	1
5) I find beauty in some things.	1	2	3	4	5	6
6) I can fit in everything I want to.	1	2	3	4	5	6
7) I feel fully mentally alert.	1	2	3	4	5	6
8) I do not have particularly happy memories of the past.	6	5	4	3	2	1

Your score: _____

SCORE INTERPRETATION

Very low levels of happiness   Super-happy

6 points ➤ 48 points

Surprised by your score? If it's lower than you'd like, don't instantly blame your GM, because, like most things, there are many factors at play. That said, hitting your gut health nutrition targets has been shown to lift your spirits. If your score is below 10, it's worth going to see your doctor for a chat. The worst thing you can do is keep it all bottled up and not tell anyone you're unhappy. People do care; I know I do. Plus, there are many support groups that can help.

Doing Damage

The impact of our lifestyle on our GM isn't always positive. Sometimes it just takes a moment for us to stop and reflect on the way we treat our bodies (and therefore our microbes), to realize that perhaps we haven't been the best hosts. They've been looking out for us, but have we been looking out for them?

To help strengthen your relationship with your GM, let's take a look at some of our GM's key vulnerabilities. In doing so, next time you're considering a certain behavior, perhaps you'll spare a thought to how it may also affect your microbes.

1. Medication

There is growing awareness that antibiotics (which translates to "anti-life" in Greek) not only kill the overgrown and "bad" bacteria but also harm the beneficial guys. In some people, these changes appear to be irreversible, meaning not all the good guys repopulate after the antibiotics. It's not just antibiotics we need to watch out for, either—a recent study has suggested that over a quarter of non-antibiotic medications (of the more than nine hundred tested) can potentially affect the growth of our gut microbes.[7]

Don't get me wrong, medications like antibiotics are incredibly important, but the next time your doctor explains that they may not be necessary because your infection is likely to be viral in origin (which means antibiotics won't work), it's worth reconsidering them. Similarly, if you're taking medication because it's easier than changing your lifestyle (decreasing your alcohol intake in the case of reflux, for example, or relying on sleeping pills instead of working on your sleep hygiene—check out page 175 for more on this), then it might be worth rethinking the potential harm you could be doing. That said, don't go getting too hasty—any decision regarding changing medication should be done under guidance from your healthcare team.

It's not all doom and gloom when it comes to our microbes and medication. One of the most common medications prescribed for type 2 diabetes (metformin) has recently been shown to benefit our GM. Studies have found a new mechanism by which metformin improves millions of patients' blood sugar regulation. And it's likely not alone, with several other medications suspected to target the GM in order to exert their medicinal benefit.

2. Sleep

Sleep disturbance, including both shift work sleep disorder and jet lag, is another major factor shown to disrupt our GM. This is because, like us, our GM exhibits a sleep-wake cycle, known as the circadian rhythm. Interestingly, the negative impact of sleep disturbance on our GM may explain, at least in part, the increased risk of weight gain and diabetes in people with disturbed sleep. Further still, research suggests that this relationship is bidirectional. This means that a disturbed GM may also lead to disturbed sleep. But there's some good news. One study showed that a type of probiotic improved sleep in a group of students, compared to a placebo (a fake probiotic).[8] In my practice, I've also found that simple dietary changes to boost our GM have helped many shift workers improve their sleep quality. Working on your sleep hygiene may also be worth thinking about, to ensure that not just you but your GM, too, gets the most out of pillow time.

For frequent fliers, particularly on long-haul flights, who also suffer from gut issues, check out page 157 for some pre-flight nutrition tips for your gut.

The impact of our lifestyle on our GM is not always positive. Sometimes it just takes a moment for us to stop and reflect on the way we treat our bodies (and therefore our microbes), to realize that perhaps we haven't been the best hosts—after all, they've been looking out for us, but have we been looking out for them?

Without intending to bring on "friend-guilt," but rather to help strengthen your relationship, let's take a look at some of our GM's key vulnerabilities. In doing so, next time you're considering a certain behavior, perhaps you'll spare a thought to how it may also affect your microbes.

3. Dieting

Did a crazy diet ever affect your GM? Interestingly, although our GM can change within a few days of being on an extreme diet, the overall changes that occur to the microbes following a short-term diet are not as extreme as you may think. What does happen, however, is that the new diet alters the function of these microbes, that is, what the microbes actually do and what they produce (the metabolome). Animal research suggests that the rapid weight regain that occurs with yo-yo dieting (when you seem to regain the weight in half the time it took you to lose it) may in fact be down to our GM.[9] The study not only demonstrated that mice with a previous "weight gain, weight loss" cycle were more susceptible to fast weight gain the second time around but also showed that this tendency to gain more weight could be transferred to other mice via a poop transplant. This suggests that the weight gain was because of their GM and not because of other factors like the mouse's metabolism. Now, before the "Oh no, what have I done?" feeling sets in, the researchers did also show that this tendency to regain weight rapidly could be reversed with the right nutrition (we'll discuss this in chapter 3).

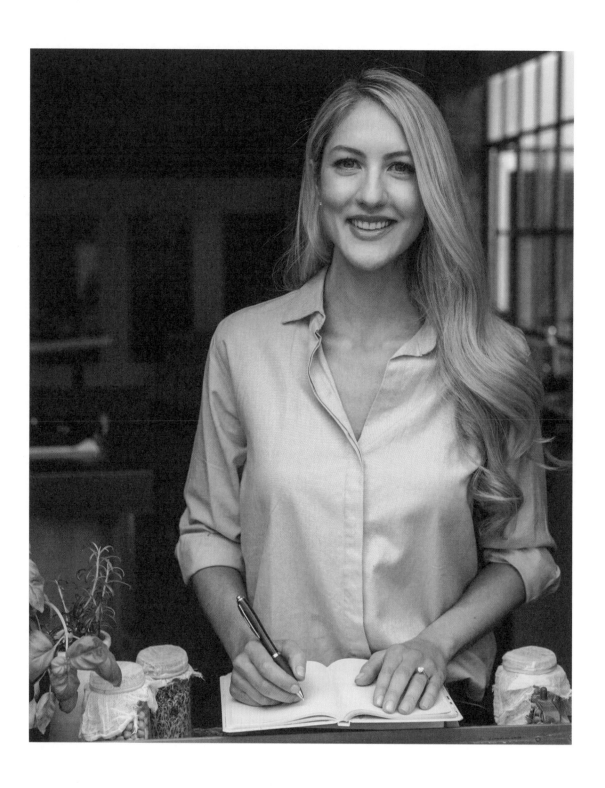

Checklist for Looking After Your GM

○ PLANT-BASED DIET DIVERSITY AND FIBER (SEE PAGE 68)

○ DON'T IGNORE GUT SYMPTOMS (SEE PAGE 89)

○ SPEND MORE TIME OUTDOORS

○ BOOST YOUR SLEEP QUALITY (SEE PAGE 175)

○ MOVE YOUR BODY OFTEN (SEE PAGE 191)

○ REDUCE YOUR STRESS LEVELS (SEE PAGE 180)

○ OPT FOR A PROBIOTIC IN SPECIFIC CASES (SEE PAGE 61)

○ AVOID UNNECESSARY MEDICATIONS AND DON'T SMOKE

○ CONSIDER A FURRY PET (CONDITIONS APPLY*)

○ TRY FERMENTED FOODS (SEE PAGE 64)

○ AVOID YO-YO DIETING

○ BE SENSIBLE WITH ALCOHOL (NO MORE THAN TWO STANDARD DRINKS A DAY)

Although research has linked furry pets with better immunity, keep in mind that pets need a lot of love and attention. If you're not up for it, just play with your neighbor's.

CHAPTER 3
Nutrition for the Gut

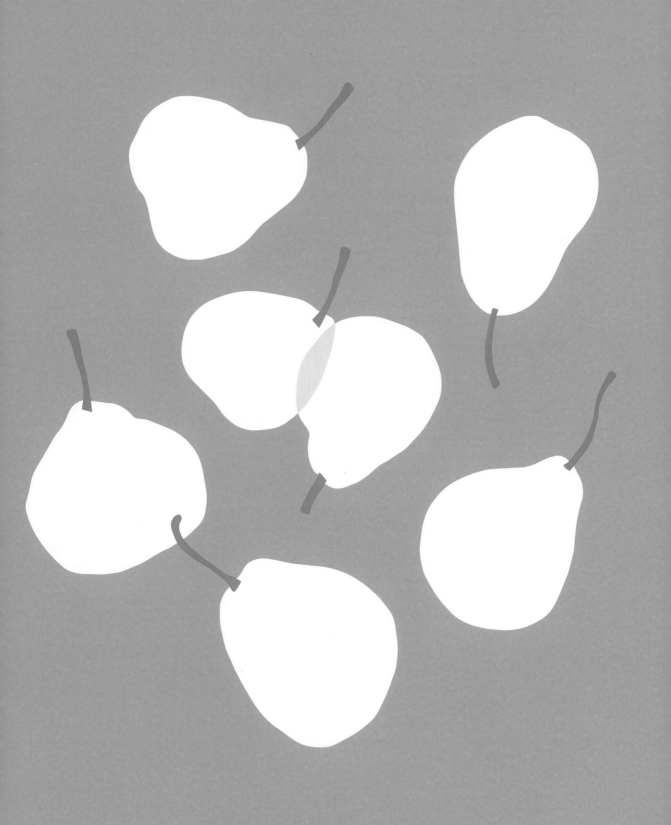

Nutrition for the Gut

It was during my PhD when I had my first ever "lightbulb moment"—one of those moments that can fundamentally alter your understanding of something. In this case, it was my understanding of nutrition. I was analyzing my patients' food diaries when it dawned on me that our view of nutrition is pretty self-centered. Mealtimes have always been about feeding ourselves: What do we want? What do we feel like eating? We rarely spare a thought for the trillions of microbes that look after us on a daily basis.

Until very recently, even the scientific community has viewed food solely through the lens of its impact on the human metabolism, forgetting completely about our GM metabolism.[10] The consequences have included some pretty drastic changes to our food supply, with the biggest one being the creation of what is now known as the "Western diet."

The Western Diet

The Western diet has been implicated in just about every chronic disease. It's characterized by excess calories; high intake of processed meats, sugary desserts, and refined grains; and high amounts of salt (think of a stereotypical fast-food meal), yet low in fiber with a limited variety of plants. We haven't always eaten like this; there was a time when we had to grow and hunt our own food and make everything from scratch. But then, in the second half of the eighteenth century, the Industrial Revolution spread across the Western world. This was the start of the downward spiral, although, at the time, the changes were thought to reflect wealth and prosperity. Food preparation moved from people's kitchens onto manufacturing lines; processed food was in, whole food was out and, as a result, daily fiber intake plummeted and added-sugar intake soared. Now, the diet has infiltrated much of the world, as industrialization increases in developing countries.

It was previously thought that fiber had no perceived nutritional benefit. Since it can't be digested by human cells, it was regarded as waste and used for animal feed (bet they had great gut health!). Indeed, up until the late twentieth century, refined grains like white bread were considered of higher quality and a marker of wealth. Thankfully, that idea has since been dismissed, although, unfortunately, the popularity of refined grains has persisted. Similarly, many food additives, such as artificial sweeteners, have increased in popularity and have been deemed safe to consume because they're not absorbed in our small intestine and therefore don't "enter" our body or directly affect human cells. But we now know that the nutrition we deliver to our microbes also plays a key role in our health and happiness.

This chapter is about rebalancing our perspective of nutrition by giving some well-deserved focus to feeding our microbes. But before we get into the real detail, let's set ourselves up by changing gear slightly and addressing any of those feelings of anxiety, stress, or even guilt that, for so many, surround the words *food* and *nutrition*. Perhaps, heading into this chapter, you were already thinking, *I wonder if I've been eating right?* or *Are my favorite foods going to be banned?* If so, I want you to get right up out of your chair, bed, or wherever you may be, and I want you to shake off those negative thoughts. Yes, that's right, I mean physically shake those shoulders and wiggle those hips. Let those negative feelings go. I know it sounds a bit absurd, but give it a try. Physically letting go of unhelpful thoughts is more powerful than you might think (something we'll discuss more in chapter 7). The fact is that nutrition is not black and white and, in my opinion, it shouldn't take precedence over the amazing flavors and feeling of community that come with eating and feeding your gut microbes. Food should be tasty, and it should be fun. Eating should be a happy experience; it shouldn't be crushed by those unhelpful thoughts, which is, sadly, something I see all too often.

One of my patients, Emily, knew all too well about the consequence of losing sight of the joy of eating. I first met Emily in my clinic six months after she'd moved away from home to start her beauty-therapy training. Emily had come to see me about her weight, which she described as "out of control." She explained, "I only have to look at food, and I gain weight these days." Emily had heard that gut inflammation was linked to weight gain and was convinced this was the cause of hers. I asked Emily to describe both her current diet and her diet six months earlier, when she had lived at home. Emily explained that she was from a family of cooks and had always loved food, but she believed that she was now paying the price for her love of fresh pasta and homemade cheese with her "inflamed" gut and resulting weight gain. Emily's current diet excluded all wheat, dairy, and foods she'd read were high in sugar; instead she ate gluten-free products, coconut oil, and vegan energy balls. When I asked her if she missed her old way of eating, she was quick to reply, "Every day! I find myself craving fresh pasta several times a week. But I know it's bad for me, and I want to look after myself." At this point, it was clear that the only way forward was to challenge some of the nutrition information Emily had heard. I started by explaining the basic functions of the gut (as we covered in chapter 1). This indirectly called into question several nutritional claims she had heard, for instance, the concept that sugar (specifically common sugar, sucrose) was bad for her GM. I showed her a diagram in an old textbook that indicated where the sugar was absorbed (in the top part of the intestine, except in very rare disorders) and explained that the small amount of sugar she had been eating was unlikely to be getting into her large intestine. Therefore, the sugar itself wasn't "harming" her GM. Instead, by restricting certain foods, such as her mom's bran cookies, which, yes, contained some sugar but also significant amounts of dietary fiber, she had actually cut down on the very nutrient that was nourishing her GM. I could see Emily starting to realize that perhaps what she'd heard wasn't all that accurate.

Toward the end of our consultation, I felt that I'd earned enough trust to propose something a little radical: For four weeks, I wanted Emily to go back to her old way of eating. That meant cooking everything from scratch, including fresh pasta (cooked al dente; I describe why on page 236), enjoying fermented dairy, and even having some of her mom's bran cookies. I also encouraged her to eat more of her meals with friends and family rather than eating alone. I could see her hesitation. But I stood by the challenge, reassuring her that I was confident her weight would not increase. Four weeks later, Emily was sitting in front of me, her weight down and her food-related quality of life up.

Why was I so confident that refocusing on the enjoyment of food would work for Emily? After eyeballing Emily's diet during our first consultation, I could see that she was not only eating much larger portions of energy-dense foods than when she had been living at home with her mom (something I commonly see when people deprive themselves of their favorite foods), she was also eating around 50 percent less fiber. Emily's case is the perfect example of how, despite good intentions, losing sight of the pleasures and feeling of community associated with eating can lead unexpectedly to negative consequences.

The good news is that nourishing your GM certainly doesn't require a strict diet, nor does it mean you have to cut out a long list of foods or give up the enjoyment of eating. In fact, part of the community feel of eating together includes feeding them, all forty trillion of them. When it comes to nutrition for your GM, it's actually pretty simple: It's just about being aware of some of the basics, like your GM's major likes and dislikes, which, I'd argue, is common courtesy, really. Think about it: Would you invite your vegan or vegetarian friends over for dinner and offer only meat? Of course not! So why not cater for our closest friends, the ones living inside our gut, which keep guard 24-7? For those after more of a scientific incentive, if you learn how to create a diet that is varied and delicious and keeps your GM happy, research suggests that you will soon see the benefits, and these go beyond kicking pesky gut symptoms, to increasing your ability to fight diseases, your happiness levels, your metabolism, and even the health of other organs, such as your heart and your liver (your main detoxing organ).

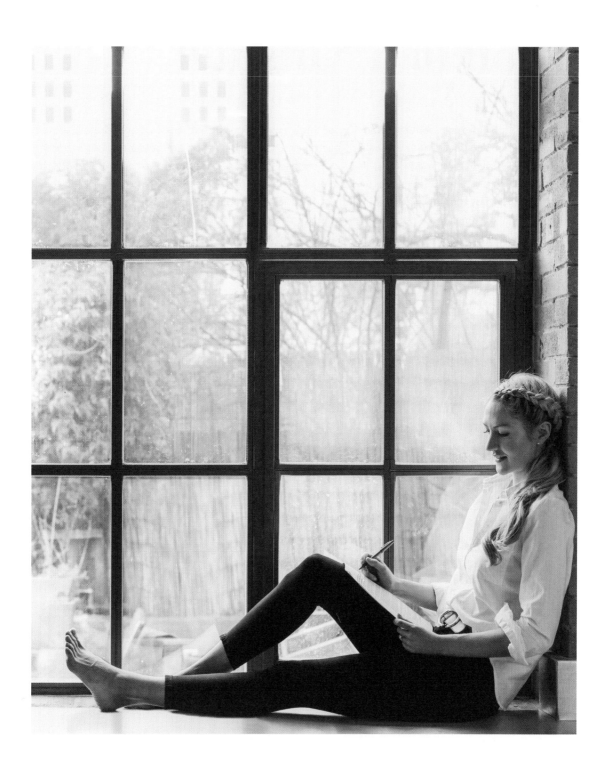

Food in a Nutshell

Food is essentially made up of three types of macronutrients: carbohydrates, proteins, and fats. These are called *macro*nutrients because they are present in large amounts, unlike *micro*nutrients, like vitamins and minerals, which are present in only very small amounts. Both macro- and micronutrients are considered essential to our diet, but they're not the only beneficial things in food. Many prebiotics and polyphenols (we'll touch on them in more detail in the pages to come) are considered food bioactives, indicating that they play an active role in our health but are not essential for basic functioning.

It's important to be aware that, at the end of the day, we eat whole foods and not single nutrients. For example, although most people refer to bread as a carbohydrate, it still contains some protein and fat. Foods are never black and white, despite our attempts to simplify and categorize them. Understanding the basics of food can help explain the big picture of diet and safeguard you against the many diet myths out there (e.g., that carb-free diets are good for your gut). With this in mind, we will start off by discussing single components of food and then tie it all together with a focus on the big picture of what we eat.

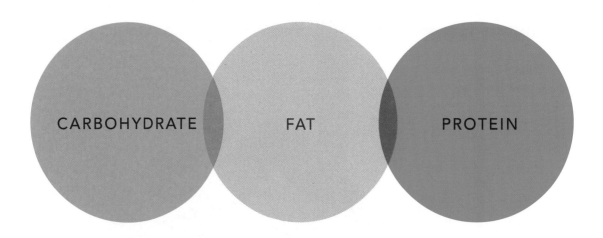

CARBOHYDRATE   FAT   PROTEIN

Macronutrients

Generally speaking, macronutrients need to be broken down into their basic building blocks before they can be absorbed from our digestive tract into our circulation: Carbohydrates are broken down into sugars, proteins into amino acids, and fat into fatty acids. This is the process of digestion, and different enzymes are required to break apart different types of macronutrients.

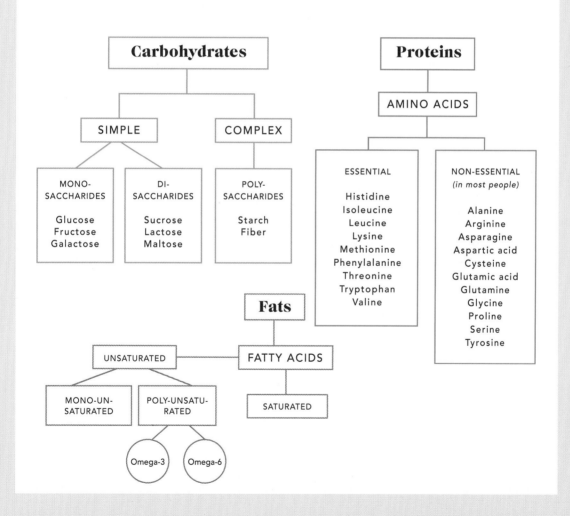

Dietary Fiber

Unlike the other types of carbohydrates (yes, fiber is a type of carbohydrate), fiber isn't broken down in the small intestine. This is because humans don't make the enzymes needed to digest it, as we touched on in chapter 1. Instead, dietary fiber continues on its merry way down the digestive tract into the large intestine, where our hungry GM eagerly awaits. I think of dietary fiber as Mother Nature's unique gift to our GM, but don't worry, we're not missing out; we get our share of the presents, as it's a mutually beneficial "transaction." Our helpful gut microbes break down many different fibers found in food, producing a range of beneficial compounds known as short-chain fatty acids (SCFA). There are three main SCFAs you may come across: acetate, propionate, and butyrate. These SCFAs are like an overachieving friend—just hearing about all the things they get up to makes you feel tired. As well as providing fuel for our gut lining, they help "get things moving" in the large intestine, contribute to the balance of blood sugars (they can trigger cells lining the intestine to make glucose, which tells our brain that we are full), stimulate our immune system and the release of gut hormones, and are also known to directly affect fat tissue, the liver, and even our brain!

The benefits of fiber don't stop there. It uses its unique physical properties to a) contribute to bulking out our poop—remember, from the Checking In with Your Poop assessment in chapter 1, a bulky poop is a good thing; b) thicken the contents of our gut, giving the gut muscles more to work with and regulating our pooping habits; and c) bind to other compounds, which can help prevent blood sugar spikes and lower cholesterol levels. If you've got an appetite for detail, check out my team's paper on all things fiber, published in one of the top science journals, *Nature Reviews*.[11]

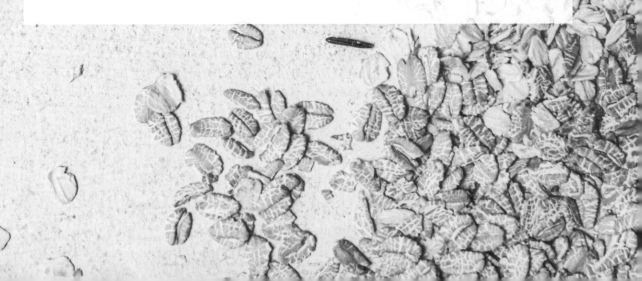

Where Do We Find It?

It's certainly no coincidence that fiber is found in the foods associated with the best health outcomes—it's essentially the backbone of plant-based foods. Each plant-based food group (whole grains, legumes, vegetables, fruits, nuts, and seeds) contains different types of fibers. In fact, there are thought to be over one hundred different types. This explains why getting fiber from different foods within each of these groups is creates the best overall health outcomes—yet another example of why diversity is key. But what if you're considering cutting out one of these groups, by going grain-free, for instance? Remember: One of my key rules is that your dietary choices are completely yours—no judgment to be found in the pages of this book. But I do want to share with you an unbiased view of the science, because a choice is only a real choice if it's an informed one.

When it comes to fiber from whole grains, there's some pretty convincing evidence for its role not just in gut health but also in reducing your chances of developing several diseases, including diabetes, heart disease, and certain cancers. In fact, according to one study involving close to sixteen thousand women, fiber from whole grains was linked with a lower risk of breast cancer, whereas fiber from vegetables and fruit didn't seem to have this benefit.[12]

Another study, this time with over four hundred thousand participants, found that those with the highest consumption of whole grains, compared to the lowest, had a reduced risk of heart issues of over 20 percent.[13] Now, this certainly doesn't mean you should be prioritizing whole grain fiber above all else, because plant-based foods are more than just fiber; they're densely packed with vitamins, minerals, polyphenols, and other bioactive components. But what it does highlight is that getting fiber from each food group is worth seriously thinking about.

How Much Do You Need?

As a general guide, when it comes to getting in your gut-boosting fibers, adults should be aiming for at least two pieces of fruit, five portions of vegetables, three portions of whole grains, and one to two portions of nuts, seeds, or legumes each day. For those into number-crunching, this will generally deliver around 30 grams of fiber, which is in line with most fiber recommendations for adults. I know this may sound like a lot, particularly with vegetables, but as you'll see in chapter 9, we've got it covered, with most of the main meal recipes providing three portions of vegetables and close to 10 grams of fiber per portion. If you'd like to up your fiber intake even further, please go right ahead. There's research that supports that going beyond 30 grams per day further lowers your risks of chronic disease like type 2 diabetes, heart disease, and depression (the SMILES trial from chapter 2 provided 50 grams per day). But before you get too heavy-handed with your fiber portions, check out my tips for the best way to increase your fiber intake on pages 58 to 59.

Lowering Your Risk

I get that, for many, making long-term changes to their diet can take a little more convincing. So here are some hard stats that I've often used with my family and friends. A powerful study has demonstrated that even small increases in fiber can have a big impact on our health. A paper published in the *Lancet*[14] (one of the top science journals) pooled together the evidence from millions of people and found that an increase of 8 grams of fiber per day was linked with:

- 19% ⬇ RISK OF HEART DISEASE

- 15% ⬇ RISK OF TYPE 2 DIABETES

- 8% ⬇ RISK OF COLON CANCER

- 7% ⬇ RISK OF DEATH FROM ALL CAUSES

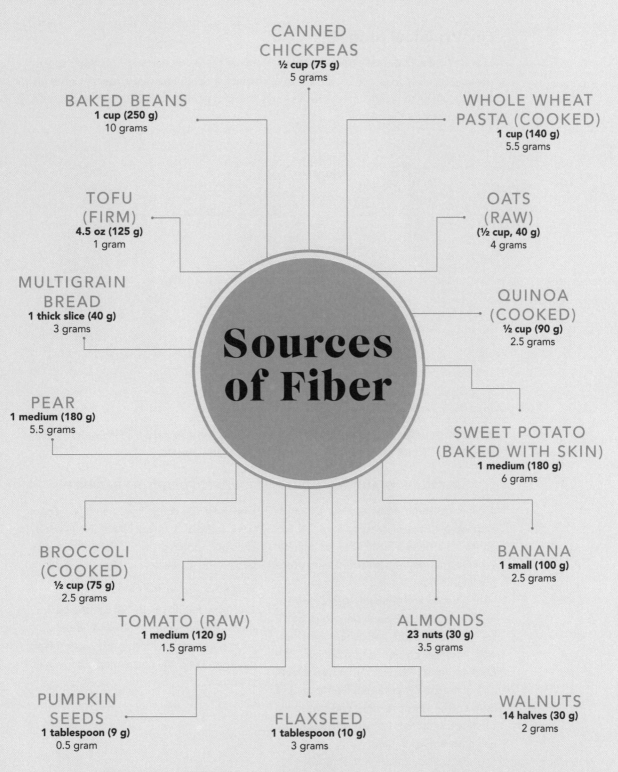

Sources of Fiber

CANNED CHICKPEAS
½ cup (75 g)
5 grams

BAKED BEANS
1 cup (250 g)
10 grams

WHOLE WHEAT PASTA (COOKED)
1 cup (140 g)
5.5 grams

TOFU (FIRM)
4.5 oz (125 g)
1 gram

OATS (RAW)
(½ cup, 40 g)
4 grams

MULTIGRAIN BREAD
1 thick slice (40 g)
3 grams

QUINOA (COOKED)
½ cup (90 g)
2.5 grams

PEAR
1 medium (180 g)
5.5 grams

SWEET POTATO (BAKED WITH SKIN)
1 medium (180 g)
6 grams

BROCCOLI (COOKED)
½ cup (75 g)
2.5 grams

BANANA
1 small (100 g)
2.5 grams

TOMATO (RAW)
1 medium (120 g)
1.5 grams

ALMONDS
23 nuts (30 g)
3.5 grams

PUMPKIN SEEDS
1 tablespoon (9 g)
0.5 gram

FLAXSEED
1 tablespoon (10 g)
3 grams

WALNUTS
14 halves (30 g)
2 grams

Source: USDA FoodData Central[15]

The Practical Stuff

As you can see, fiber really does deserve a prominent place on our plate. So, what constitutes a portion of fiber-rich food? Not to get fanatical about measuring food—I certainly don't recommend weighing your meals—but having a general idea of what constitutes a portion is helpful. So here it is:

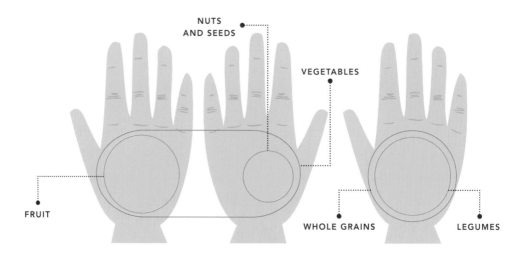

NUTS AND SEEDS

VEGETABLES

FRUIT

WHOLE GRAINS

LEGUMES

WHEN IT COMES TO INCREASING THE AMOUNT OF PLANT-BASED FOODS IN OUR DIET, THERE ARE THREE THINGS WORTH KNOWING:

1. INCREASE SLOW AND GRADUALLY

It takes our large intestine time to adjust and adapt to the increased "load." If you go from a little to a lot of fiber too quickly, your GM may get a little carried away (think post-diet binge), leaving your gut feeling a little bloated and probably gassy, too. To avoid this, start by increasing your intake by one portion per day. After one week, add another portion and continue this gradual pattern of weekly increases until you've reached your target. If your gut is a little on the sensitive side, you might like to start a little more slowly, increasing by half a portion each time.

2. DON'T FORGET TO HYDRATE

Generally speaking, fiber needs water to work some of its magic. With this in mind, consider adding an extra glass of water or two as you increase your fiber-rich foods.

3. MAKE THEM IRRESISTIBLE

Changing habits can be hard at the best of times, so help yourself out and "dress up" your plant-based foods with tasty flavor combos. We'll be doing plenty of this in chapter 9.

Ways to Boost Your Fiber Intake

1

Add flavor and texture to your favorite soup by stirring in cooked barley or legumes.

2

Sprinkle mixed seeds on your breakfast—whether it's cereal, toast, or eggs, it's always a winner.

3

Love meat lasagna? Why not replace a third of the ground meat with cooked lentils for a twist your GM will love, too?

4

Don't waste your time or fiber—keep the skin on your fruit and vegetables.

5

Baking muffins? Replace one third of the flour with quick oats.

6

Up the fiber in your take-out and add a side portion of vegetables or mixed salad with whatever you're having.

7

Add low-sugar granola to your yogurt—a delicious crunch with no cooking necessary.

8

Boost your Bolognese sauce by adding lentils or legumes, or by grating in onion, carrots, and zucchini.

9

Making meatballs? Replace a third of the meat with uncooked oats, lentils, or legumes.

10

In a rush? Frozen vegetables are a convenient and nutritious addition to any meal.

11

Banish those hungry feelings with a small handful of nuts, seeds, and dried fruit.

12

Make the switch from white to whole-grain and seeded bread—your GM will thank you.

Prebiotics

A *prebiotic*—not to be mistaken for a *probiotic*—is food that feeds specific beneficial microbes. But wait, isn't that the same as fiber? Indeed, most prebiotics are a type of dietary fiber, although not all dietary fibers are prebiotics. There are two reasons for this. First, not all fibers can be eaten by our GM. Second, for a dietary fiber to "win" a prebiotic title, it must prove itself in several scientific trials, meaning it really does have to work for that coveted prebiotic title.

The main prebiotics include inulin, fructo-oligosaccharides (FOS), and galacto-oligo-saccharides (GOS). These are found in over 35,000 plant species, with some of the most common sources listed below. The benefits of prebiotics range from improving blood sugar control and appetite regulation to supporting bone health and skin health. There are also a number of trials demonstrating the benefit of prebiotics on immunity, with some pretty convincing evidence that prebiotics can reduce your risk of needing antibiotics, particularly in children and the elderly.

So, which prebiotic supplement do I recommend you take? It's simple: none. That's right: For the majority of people, taking advantage of the naturally occurring prebiotics in food is absolutely the best way to feed your GM. There are some scenarios in which I do recommend supplements, but these are infrequent and should be considered on a case-by-case basis. If you are considering taking a prebiotic supplement, keep in mind that more is not always better.

Fruit	Vegetables	Grains & nuts	Others
Apricots	Artichokes	Almonds	Black tea
Dates	Asparagus	Amaranth	Chamomile tea
Dried figs	Beets	Barley	Dandelion tea
Dried mango	Brussels sprouts	Cashews	Fennel tea
Grapefruit	Chicory root	Freekeh	Green tea
Nectarines	Fennel bulb	Hazelnuts	Legumes
Persimmons	Garlic	Pistachios	(black beans,
Pomegranates	Leeks	Rye	butter beans,
Prunes	Okra	Spelt	chickpeas, etc.)
Watermelon	Onions	Wheat berries	Quince paste
			Silken tofu

Probiotics

Next up is probiotics, which is the term used to describe microbes that are good for us; they're the ones we want in our gut. Now, just like the term prebiotic, *probiotic is a title that a microbe must earn. It's also worth keeping in mind that, although most common probiotics are a type of bacteria, some are also yeast.*

THERE ARE THREE MAIN CRITERIA TO FULFILL THE PROBIOTIC DEFINITION:

1. THE MICROBES HAVE TO BE ALIVE.

2. THEY HAVE TO BE PRESENT IN LARGE NUMBERS.

3. THEY HAVE TO HAVE EVIDENCE OF A HEALTH BENEFIT.

Who Should Take a Probiotic Capsule?

Generally speaking, if you're in good health, the evidence for taking a probiotic at this stage is actually pretty weak. If there's something in particular that you're aiming to manage (a gut symptom or a health condition, for example), then, in some cases, it may be advisable. It all comes down to your specific condition and whether there is any evidence for a particular type of probiotic. It's also worth recognizing that different probiotics do different things and therefore have different indications. It's like medication—you wouldn't take a painkiller to improve your cholesterol. One of my patients, Hayley, is a good example of this.

Hayley came to see me after suffering for several years with IBS. She had previously tried the standard dietary recommendations for IBS (we'll discuss them in chapter 6), and although that did improve some of her symptoms, she was traveling frequently for work and found them difficult to implement consistently. Hayley had continued living with her bothersome bloating, belly cramps, and loose poops until she had an "accident" at work. When I asked Hayley if she was taking any supplements, she explained that she'd tried several probiotics that her friends had recommended but hadn't found any that helped her. Hayley was excited to give one of the clinically backed probiotics a try. We matched the particular type of bacteria, the dose, and the duration. Hayley documented her symptoms for seven days before she started taking them and then again four weeks after.

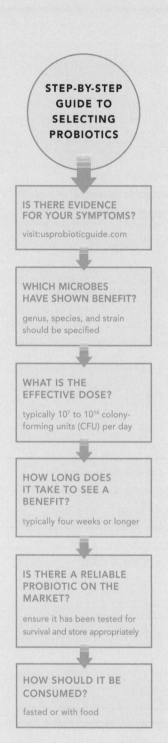

STEP-BY-STEP GUIDE TO SELECTING PROBIOTICS

IS THERE EVIDENCE FOR YOUR SYMPTOMS?

visit:usprobioticguide.com

WHICH MICROBES HAVE SHOWN BENEFIT?

genus, species, and strain should be specified

WHAT IS THE EFFECTIVE DOSE?

typically 10^7 to 10^{14} colony-forming units (CFU) per day

HOW LONG DOES IT TAKE TO SEE A BENEFIT?

typically four weeks or longer

IS THERE A RELIABLE PROBIOTIC ON THE MARKET?

ensure it has been tested for survival and store appropriately

HOW SHOULD IT BE CONSUMED?

fasted or with food

Strain: the type of probiotic, i.e., microbe, shown to have a benefit. **CFU:** colony-forming units. This is the unit that bacteria are measured in, similar to how protein is measured in grams.

Three weeks into Hayley's trial, I received an email from her describing the positive impact the probiotics were having, not only on her symptoms but also on her anxiety (which I saw as very much linked with her symptoms). But she wasn't just emailing about the good news; Hayley had a urinary tract infection and was prescribed antibiotics. She had taken them before and said that they'd messed with her gut, so she was worried they'd undo all the good work that had come from the probiotics. I suggested that she stop taking her IBS probiotics and instead replace them with a probiotic designed specifically to help prevent antibiotic-associated gut upset (known as antibiotic-associated diarrhea, which we'll discuss on page 100), a common side effect of antibiotics. When I saw Hayley in the clinic two weeks later, her symptoms had continued to improve and she was thrilled to report that the antibiotics had only a minimal impact on her symptoms. Although Hayley acknowledged that there were still some lifestyle changes she needed to make, finding a probiotic that worked for her gave her the confidence boost she needed to persist.

When deciding whether a probiotic is right for you, there are several things worth considering. To help simplify things, I've summarized the six steps I recommend you follow in the graphic on this page. As a guide to get you started, I have also developed a summary of evidence-based probiotic prescriptions opposite.

Probiotic Prescriptions

To help you get the most out of this new area, I've developed a guide, in collaboration with my colleagues, describing the probiotic prescriptions you may like to consider for conditions where there is a body of evidence (i.e., there has been a supportive meta-analysis) suggesting at least some benefit. When considering taking a probiotic, it's worth keeping in mind that even the area with the most convincing evidence (antibiotic-associated diarrhea), following the prescription still doesn't guarantee it will work for you—it's up to you to weigh the risk (typically financial cost) versus the benefit. If you are interested in giving it a try, remember to assess what you're looking to change (e.g., a symptom) before and then again after taking the probiotic for the duration outlined below. This way you can get a more objective idea of whether it's worth your time and money.

Condition	Prescription*
Irritable bowel syndrome (for overall symptoms, including tummy pain, bloating, and flatulence)	**Strain:** *Lactobacillus plantarum* 299v **Dose:** 10 billion CFU per day **Form:** Capsule **Duration:** 4 weeks **Timing:** Daily**
Antibiotic-associated diarrhea	**Strain:** a) *Lactobacillus rhamnosus* GG or b) *Saccharomyces boulardii* **Dose:** a) 6 billion CFU, twice per day; b) 5 billion CFU, twice per day **Form:** Powder **Duration:** While taking antibiotics, plus for an additional week after **Timing:** 2 hours after breakfast and dinner
Constipation	**Strain:** a) *Lactobacillus plantarum* LP01 and *Bifidobacterium breve* BR03; or b) *Bifidobacterium lactis* BS01 **Dose:** 5 billion CFU per day **Form:** Powder **Duration:** 4 weeks **Timing:** First thing in the morning
Respiratory tract infections (e.g., common cold)	**Strain:** *Lactobacillus rhamnosus* GG and *Bifidobacterium lactis* BB-12 **Dose:** 2 billion CFU per day **Form:** Powder **Duration:** 12 weeks **Timing:** Once daily
H. pylori infection (stomach infection) (alongside antibiotic therapy)	**Strain:** Lactobacillus acidophilus LA-5 and *Bifidobacterium lactis* BB-12 **Dose:** 5 billion CFU, twice per day **Form:** 7 ounces (200 g) yogurt **Duration:** 1 week (while taking antibiotics) and 4 weeks post-antibiotics **Timing:** 30 minutes after antibiotic, twice per day
Preventing eczema in babies with a parent who has eczema	**Strain:** *Lactobacillus rhamnosus* HN001 **Dose:** 6 billion CFU per day **Form:** mother: capsule; baby: powder **Duration:** mother: from 35 weeks of pregnancy to 6 months postpartum (if breastfeeding); baby: from 6 days to 2 years old **Timing:** Once daily
Ulcerative colitis (inducing remission in mild to moderately active, alongside standard medical therapy)	**Strains:** 8-strain combination Visbiome: 4 strains of *Lactobacilli* (*L. paracasei, L. plantarum, L. acidophilus*, and *L. delbrueckii* subsp. *bulgaricus*): 3 strains of *Bifidobacteria* (*B. longum, B. infantis, B. breve*); 1 strain of *Streptococcus thermophilus.* **Dose:** 1.8 trillion CFU, twice per day*** **Form:** Powder, mixed with cold water or yogurt **Duration:** 12 weeks **Timing:** Morning and evening
Hayfever (allergic rhinitis) (alongside antihistamine)	**Strain:** *Lactobacillus paracasei* LP-33 **Dose:** 2 billion CFU per day **Form:** Capsule **Duration:** 5 weeks along with loratadine (antihistamine), plus an additional 2 weeks **Timing:** With food

*Based on one placebo-controlled trial; additional probiotic strains have also shown benefit. See usprobioticguide.com.

**Sometimes studies don't give the exact detail of when the probiotic was taken (i.e., time and whether it's with food). In such cases, follow the instructions on the product label.

***This isn't a typo. This prescription is at a much higher dose than others. There were no safety issues found in the study, other than 18 percent of the probiotic group reporting some bloating in the first few days, which resolved within a week.[16]

Fermented Foods

Let me start by declaring that I am pro-fermented-food—the flavors, the journey, and the (albeit anecdotal) health benefits associated with them have earned them a regular place in my diet. But with my science hat on, I must admit that the concept of a fermented food and its health benefits are not as straightforward as you may have hoped.

Despite their recent rise in popularity, fermented foods have been around for thousands of years. In fact, fermented food has earned a prized place in most cultures, each crafting unique flavors and traditions around the art of fermenting. Some of my favorites include Japanese natto (soybeans), Korean kimchi (usually cabbage), Slavic kvass (a non-alcoholic rye drink), French crème fraîche (soured cream), Mexican *pozol* (a corn drink), Ethiopian injera (teff flatbread), Indian *dhokla* (steamed breakfast cakes), Indonesian tempeh (soybean cake), just to name a few. . . .

Generally speaking, any food or drink that relies on microbes to convert simple ingredients into a final product fits the fermented-food bill. Indeed, as much as one third of our daily diet is thought to rely on the process of fermentation: bread, chocolate, cheese, yogurt, olives, vinegar, soy sauce, coffee, and even alcohol. Now, before you blame last weekend's cocktail binge on a selfless quest for good gut health, fermented doesn't automatically mean it's good for you. Similarly, not all fermented food contains live microbes. This is because many die off in the making, during processes involving heat (e.g., in the case of bread) and filtration (e.g., in the case of wine). Nonetheless, the benefits of fermented food extend beyond the live microbes. This has been observed with sourdough bread: Even though the microbes die off during baking, when compared to unfermented whole wheat bread, the sourdough had a better effect on blood sugars. Now I must declare that this was just a single study,[17] so not to be taken as gospel. Similarly, although not all yogurts contain significant amounts of live microbes, yogurt has been linked with more pronounced health benefits in large studies,[18] including weight management, compared to unfermented dairy products such as milk.

On the whole, the scientific evidence behind fermented foods is limited.[19] But this certainly shouldn't be interpreted as saying that eating fermented foods has no benefit (anecdotally speaking, I believe many do); it's just that the high-quality studies in humans haven't been done yet—something I'm passionate about changing. Health benefits aside, many traditional forms of fermented food are delicious, so why not give them a try? For a beginner's guide to making your own fermented foods, as well as the practical aspects, such as how much you should be having, head to page 290.

Potential Benefits of Traditional Fermented Foods

Each benefit is unique to different fermented foods.

1. CONTAIN LIVE MICROBES linked with a wide range of health benefits (check out their résumé on page 35).

2. IMPROVE TASTE, TEXTURE, AND DIGESTIBILITY (e.g., fermentation of grape skins enhances the extraction of those gut-loving polyphenols found in red wine). Fermenting may also lower the gluten content in some sourdough breads, and lactose (milk sugar) in dairy products.

3. CAN INCREASE CONCENTRATIONS OF VITAMINS such as folate, riboflavin, and B_{12}.

4. CONTAIN BENEFICIAL COMPOUNDS such as organic acids, which may help to reduce blood pressure, improve blood sugar control, and support the immune system. Brain-messenger molecules such as gamma-aminobutyric acids (GABA), which are known to have a calming effect on the brain, are also found in some fermented food.

5. MAY REMOVE/REDUCE TOXINS AND ANTINUTRIENTS (e.g., fermentation can significantly reduce phytic acid, which, although not harmful per se, can inhibit the absorption of other nutrients such as zinc, as we discuss on page 77).

Phytochemicals

Phytochemicals is just the sciencey name for a group of plant chemicals. As we touched on earlier, these are different from macronutrients (e.g., fats and protein) and micronutrients (e.g., folate and iron) because they're not essential. Instead, consider them as a way to boost your health a little bit further. It's kind of like buying a new pair of sneakers or new model of phone—neither is essential, but both can enhance your performance and efficiency. One of the most well-studied classes of phytochemical is the polyphenols. These include flavanols, which are linked to the health benefits of dark chocolate, and anthocyanin, which gives berries their brilliant red, purple, and blue color. Around 90 percent of polyphenols are malabsorbed in the small intestine and therefore join our GM in the large intestine. This is where much of the magic is thought to happen, in that our microbes help to transform them into a range of absorbable and potentially beneficial chemicals linked with cancer prevention and better heart and mental health.

Things get even more fascinating. The benefits of polyphenols appear to be dependent on your unique GM and whether it's able to metabolize the specific polyphenol you've eaten. My colleagues at King's College London are currently investigating whether this GM-dependency may explain why some people do better on different diets.

So where can we find these health boosters? Polyphenols are found in a wide range of plant-based foods, with some of the top sources outlined in the following graphic. It's worth thinking about how many make a regular appearance in your diet. Are there any you might like to try? To get more into your diet, why not add some berries to your breakfast bowl, or olives to your pasta sauce, or hazelnuts to your salad? For those tempted to reach for the supplement instead, consider that, in most cases, the polyphenols found in whole foods are linked with the best health outcomes.

We often forget the power of herbs and spices, but not only do they add even more polyphenols to your diet, they can seriously boost the flavor of your meals. You might like to experiment with the top polyphenol-containing seasonings on the opposite page.

Top Polyphenol Foods

- **DRINKS**
  Filtered coffee, black tea, red wine, green tea, cocoa

- **FRUIT**
  Blueberry, black currant, plum, cherry, blackberry, strawberry, raspberry, prune, apple

- **NUTS AND SEEDS**
  Flaxseed, chestnuts, hazelnuts, pecans, almonds

- **VEGETABLES AND LEGUMES**
  Black olives, green olives, globe artichoke heads, roasted soybeans, chicories, red onion, spinach, black beans, white beans, broccoli, asparagus

- **FATS**
  Extra virgin olive oil, canola oil

Top fifteen herbs & spices			
	• CAPERS	• OREGANO	• BASIL
	• CELERY SEEDS	• PEPPERMINT	• CURRY POWDER
	• CLOVES	• ROSEMARY	• GINGER
	• SAGE	• SPEARMINT	• CINNAMON
	• THYME	• STAR ANISE	• CARAWAY SEEDS

Source: European Journal of Clinical Nutrition[20]
(Ranked per 100 g.) Values can differ between crops.

Plant-Based Diet Diversity

According to the United Nations, 75 percent of plant diversity has been lost since the 1900s, resulting in today's comparatively limited range of plant-based foods. This alarming loss is the consequence of farmers having been forced to ditch their local varieties for genetically uniform, high-yield crops to keep up with society's demand for "perfect" food. Think about the way you shop. Do you always reach for those shiny, red, extra-sweet apples, or do you go for the odd-shaped ones with color imperfections? I was certainly a shiny-red-apple kind of shopper—until I found out that often the types that were exposed to more stressful growing conditions (resulting in imperfections) contain more polyphenols. I now hunt for and celebrate those imperfections. Perhaps the same principle applies to our own life, too. Now there's some food for thought.

In terms of our overall diet diversity, it gets worse, with 75 percent of the world's food being generated from only twelve plant and five animal species. Essentially, this means that both our taste buds and our GM are missing out on so many foods. The consequence? This restricted diet is thought to starve microbes that require a diverse nutrient supply, and may very well explain why, compared to our ancestors, our GM diversity as a population has taken quite the hit. I think we can do better, don't you?

> TAKE-HOME MESSAGE: *The more diversity in your plant-based diet, the more diverse the nutrient supply for your GM (think dietary fibers, prebiotics, and polyphenols). All in all, this equates to a well-fed and diverse range of happy gut microbes, each with their own unique skill set to complement ours.*

So where do you start? It's very much up to you. If you're still working on getting in your minimum daily portion of plant-based foods (two pieces of fruit; five portions of vegetables; three portions of whole grains; and one or two portions of nuts, seeds, or legumes), don't get overwhelmed by the thought of adding diversity into the mix—stick with the foods you're comfortable with. Once you're feeling confident, or if you've already got those portions down and want that extra boost, this is where diversity comes into play. My motto: Aim for thirty plant points a week across all plant-based food groups (that's thirty different fruits, vegetables, whole grains, legumes, nuts and seeds, herbs, and spices). It quickly adds up and is easier than you may think!

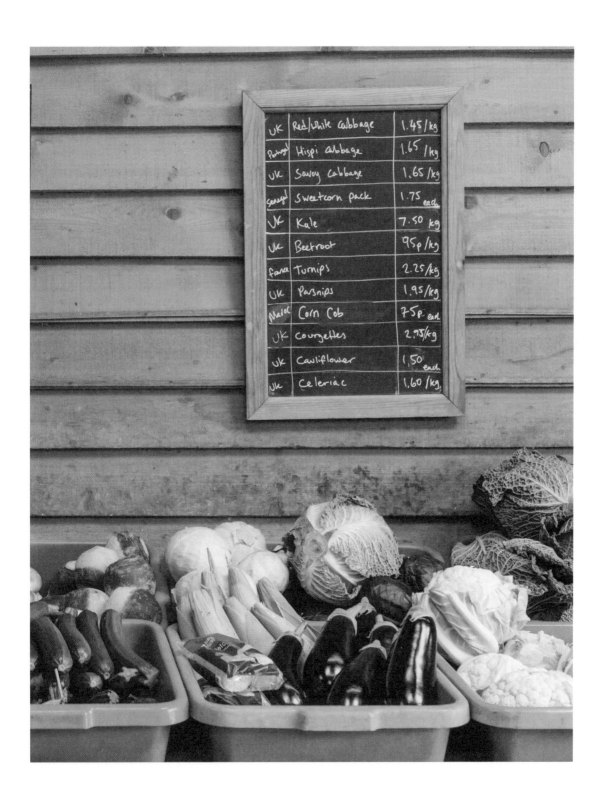

Food Form

It's not just about what foods we eat—it's also about the food's form. The physical structure of a food can affect digestion. For example, my colleagues have demonstrated that, compared to instant oats (the ones that turn to oatmeal in two minutes), large, steel-cut oats had a 33 percent lower effect on blood sugar levels. This means the sugars were digested more slowly—they had a lower glycemic index, or GI. This suggests that the large, less processed versions of foods are probably better for blood sugar management, preventing sugar spikes.

What About the Health of the Environment?

The good news is that prioritizing plant-based foods is much less taxing on the planet, too. In fact, gas emissions caused by a vegetarian diet are almost 50 percent lower than those caused by meat eaters. If the thought of cutting meat out is a little intimidating, don't worry, I hear you. Start by making small changes—cutting down your intake (below 3.5 ounces/100 g per day) still reduces your carbon footprint by over 20 percent.

Top five switch-and-saves on your carbon footprint		
THIS ... FOR ... THAT		CARBON-FOOTPRINT SAVING
BEEF (26.5)	legumes (0.5) (see recipe on page 260)	98%
CHEESE (8.5)	cashew cheese (1.5) (see recipe on page 237)	83%
BUTTER (9.5)	avocado (1.5)	86%
CREAM (5.5)	yogurt (1.5) (see recipe on page 306)	77%
LAMB (25.5)	tofu (1.0) (see recipe on page 250)	96%

Source: Journal for Cleaner Production[21]
(Kilograms of greenhouse gases/kilogram of food)

Fasting

To fast or not to fast? Although there is evidence from animal studies that intermittent fasting may benefit our metabolism via its impact on our GM, there is little evidence from human studies to date. There are two main types of intermittent fasting: alternate-day fasting (such as the 5:2 diet, where you consume less than 600 calories on two days and eat normally on the other five days of the week) and time-restricted fasting (such as the 16:8 diet, where you limit your intake to an eight-hour daily eating "window" and fast for the remaining sixteen hours). It is true that these types of diets, when followed, can help with weight management, simply because you have less opportunity to eat and therefore your total food intake is reduced. If you're overweight, losing weight can have many health benefits. These include lowering blood pressure and blood fats, improving your blood sugar regulation, and lowering your risk of (or even reversing) type 2 diabetes. There is also some early-stage evidence that eating in alignment with our circadian rhythm has benefits, independent of weight loss. More specifically, increasing our food intake at breakfast (when our body appears to be better primed for food) and reducing it in the evening may improve our body's blood sugar regulation, even if we don't lose weight. However, as with most diets, they can be difficult to sustain beyond a month or two, and they can affect not only our relationship with food but our mood, too (no one enjoys being hungry!). That said, I believe it's very much an individualized approach. It may suit some people, but it's just not something I'd recommend to everyone without there being strong evidence behind it. If you are interested in intermittent fasting, why not start by decreasing your current eating window by just an hour on either side and see how it feels for you? And if you do want to go the whole way, here are some things to consider: 1) Ensure you're still meeting your daily fiber needs—your microbes don't like to starve either; 2) if you have IBS, aim to spread your meals out as much as possible and avoid large meals, as we'll discuss in chapter 6; and 3) if you take regular medication, check with your doctor beforehand, as it may affect how they function.

Additional Nutrients

This is where things can get a little more complicated. We now know nutrition is certainly not black and white and, no surprise, neither is digestion. It's worth noting that some nutrients, such as protein and fat, can escape digestion in the small intestine and make its way into the large intestine. So it makes sense that they, too, can affect the happiness of our GM, particularly if we overconsume. Like us, our GM is able to digest a wide range of nutrients, so it can survive—well, a core number of microbes, anyway—on pretty much whatever we throw at it. However, there's a vital difference between surviving and thriving. Too many of these nutrients in the large intestine may have some unfavorable side effects. Take protein, for instance. Excess intake can not only result in foul-smelling gas (those who've succumbed to a high-protein diet will know what I mean), but it's also thought to give rise to a more aggressive GM environment, sometimes likened to the concept of "roid rage." When our microbes ferment too much protein, they release chemical compounds that have been associated with damaging health outcomes, which have been implicated in colon cancer and inflammatory bowel disease. More recently, a trial has shown that protein supplementation for ten weeks resulted in a decrease in several health-promoting bacteria, and another study showed a reduction in the beneficial short-chain fatty acid (SCFA) butyrate. Further, my and others' research suggests that what may be more important than total protein is the ratio of protein to fiber. This means that if you eat lots of protein (from large portions of animal products) but also lots of fiber,[22] the negative impact on your GM is likely reduced. So, if you do enjoy those high-protein animal foods, try to eat them with fiber-rich foods, including whole grains, vegetables and legumes, and herbs and spices.

There isn't a great deal of research looking specifically at fat and our microbes. What we do know is that the Mediterranean diet contains around 40 percent fat and is associated with high GM diversity. Yet other high-fat diets such as the Western diet with a similar ratio of fat are associated with lower GM diversity. This is yet another reason why fixating on individual nutrients is likely unhelpful; it's more about the type of foods you choose. For example, whole wheat sourdough dipped in extra virgin olive oil is going to be a better option than deep-fried potato wedges dipped in ketchup, although the two are equivalent in fat percentage.

What About Omega-3?

This type of fat, found in oily fish such as salmon and in plant sources such as walnuts and flaxseeds, has been shown to increase SCFA-producing bacteria such as *Roseburia*. Perhaps the gut-brain axis we touched on in chapter 2 may also explain, at least in part, the link between omega-3 and improvement in mood disorders. With this in mind, here are five recipes that can help you boost your omega-3 intake.

Five Recipes to Boost Your Omega-3 Intake

1 QUINOA SUSHI ROLLS (PAGE 243)

2 LEMON CURD TARTLETS WITH A CHIA AND CASHEW CRUST (PAGE 282)

3 RAW CARROT CAKE BALLS (PAGE 278)

4 SATAY TOFU SKEWERS WITH SAUCY GREENS (PAGE 250)

5 CHEESY VEGAN CRACKERS (PAGE 269)

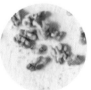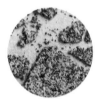

Food Additives

Artificial sweeteners, including sucralose and aspartame, are among the most widely used food additives today, but is there really such a thing as a free meal? Here's the thing: All additives must undergo a rigorous safety assessment before they're allowed to be included in our food supply. But historically, the safety assessments haven't considered the impact on our GM—because a lot of these assessments were undertaken before we had a grasp on the importance of it. Some early studies (most are in animals, not humans) demonstrate that certain types of artificial sweeteners (such as sucralose, saccharin, and aspartame) negatively affect the GM, promoting blood sugar issues, liver inflammation, and weight gain.[23] Furthermore, animal studies have supported a causal relationship, showing that these negative consequences can be transferred between mice via a poop transplant.[24] But it's worth knowing that only a subset of the results from animal studies actually translates in humans. In human studies of the effects of artificial sweeteners, there are conflicting findings: Some suggest they're beneficial (as an alternative to added sugar), while others suggest they're not so good. This is likely explained by the fact that we all house different microbes that can respond differently. This is illustrated by a very small but important study that showed that daily intake of saccharin at a dose in line with the high end of the "safe" amount (a level set by health authorities) for one week negatively affected the blood sugar of only a small subset of people. So, when it comes to artificial sweeteners and their impact on your gut microbes, the jury is still out.[25]

Other additives, including a group known as emulsifiers, which are found in a wide range of processed foods (particularly frozen desserts, cakes, and cookies), have also been implicated in triggering prediabetes and gut inflammation, at least in mice. My research team is looking to get to the bottom of this with the world's first food-additive trial, to look at the impact of food additives on gut inflammation in people with IBD. I'll be sure to keep you updated.

Salt (Sodium Chloride)

Salt is added to most processed food in large amounts. Around 75 percent of the salt we eat is in processed foods, including breakfast cereals, instant soups, processed meats, snacks like chips and cookies, and prepared foods. Foods containing more than 1.5 grams of salt or 0.6 grams of sodium per 100 grams are considered high in salt. High salt intake can lead to high blood pressure, which may lead to heart disease, and emerging research suggests that our GM may also play an active role in this process. Indeed, a high-quality human study demonstrated that reducing salt intake led to an increase in those beneficial SCFA (particularly in females), which are thought to be involved in the regulation of blood pressure (yet another talent of theirs[26]). There have been a number of trials investigating the role of probiotics as a therapy for high blood pressure. Although most have found a small improvement, overall, the size of the benefit means it's probably not worth your money at this point. For now, try the tips below to help reduce your salt intake.

1. CUT THE HABIT
Refill your saltshaker on the dinner table with pepper and mixed herbs.

2. TAKE IT SLOWLY
Reducing salt gradually over a few months allows your taste buds to adapt and become more sensitive to salt.

3. SAY NO TO PREMADE SAUCES
Instead, experiment with fresh herbs and spices to bring out the flavors in your dish (see page 67 for inspiration).

Piecing It All Together

OK, so what does the ultimate gut-health diet look like? The truth is, there is no single gut-health diet. There are, however, guiding principles that underpin an eating pattern that supports good gut health. If you only take one thing away, this is it: The power of plant diversity is key, and the more the merrier. What this looks like in terms of final foods is really up to you, your preferences, and where you are on your gut health journey. This same concept is observed within the "Blue Zones"—five regions around the world where people live particularly long and healthy lives. Despite sharing several fundamental principles, including a focus on plant-based foods, many aspects of their diet, including intake of dairy and meat, are inconsistent, with some zones including them and others not. This reinforces the fact that there is no single "right" way to eat. That said, if you are cutting out entire food groups, you're naturally at an increased risk of a nutritional deficiency. Rest assured: It is possible to get all the nutrients you need from other foods. For instance, in some cultures that limit dairy, people consume calcium-rich bony fish and make the most of non-dietary factors that affect bone health, such as getting enough vitamin D from the sun and doing weight-bearing exercises. If the nutritional adequacy of your diet is in doubt, it is best to discuss it with your dietitian or registered nutritionist.

Specific Nutrients to Consider If You're Eating a Purely Plant-Based Diet

Calcium: Dairy foods are rich in calcium. If you're not eating these, choose calcium-fortified plant-based milks. Other sources include tofu (check on the label that it's set with calcium chloride or calcium sulphate), sardines or salmon with bones, and spring greens. Keep in mind that, although spinach contains calcium, it's mostly bound to a compound called oxalate, which limits its absorption.

Iodine: Seafood is a good source of iodine. If you don't eat seafood, you may like to consider including sea vegetables in your diet (try the Quinoa Sushi Rolls on page 243). While plant-based foods such as cereals and grains can be a source of iodine, the levels vary depending on the amount of iodine in the soil where the plants were grown.

Iron: The iron found in plants (nonheme iron) is less efficiently absorbed. To help your body absorb iron from plant foods, include a source of vitamin C with your meals. These include tomatoes, peppers, oranges, and strawberries.

Omega-3 Fats: Most of the health benefits of omega-3 have been linked to animal-based sources (docosahexaenoic acid, or DHA, and eicosapentaenoic acid, or EPA). The plant-based type of omega-3 (alpha-linolenic acid, or ALA) can be converted by our bodies into DHA and EPA. But the conversion is not efficient, which is why, if you're vegan, it's important to include plenty of the plant-based sources, as discussed on page 73, and consider fortified foods or supplements.

Selenium: Meat, fish, and nuts are good sources of selenium. If you're purely plant-based, it's best to include nuts in your diet. Brazil nuts top the selenium charts.

Vitamin B$_{12}$: Eggs and dairy are good sources of B$_{12}$. If you're vegan, consider foods fortified with B$_{12}$, including fortified plant-based milks and yogurts. Nutritional yeast is another source, which I commonly use in cooking for its cheesy flavor profile. Check out my Cashew Cheese (page 237).

Zinc: Phytates found in plant foods such as whole grains and legumes can reduce zinc absorption. Fermenting (see page 290) and sprouting (see page 293) can help reduce the amount of phytates in these foods. Nuts and seeds are also good sources.

Gut Health on a Plate

As a starting guide, I've plated an example below of what good gut-health eating might look like. This reflects my seven guiding principles (opposite) that support good gut health. Remember: This is just a guide for you to tweak according to your (and your microbes') preferences.

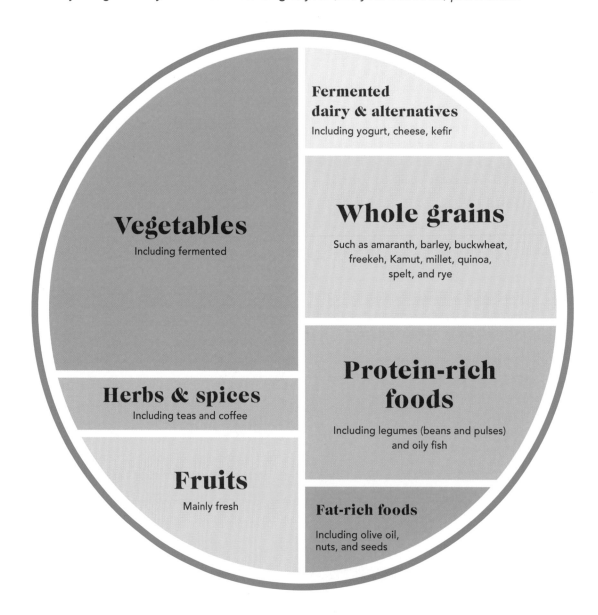

Fermented dairy & alternatives
Including yogurt, cheese, kefir

Vegetables
Including fermented

Whole grains
Such as amaranth, barley, buckwheat, freekeh, Kamut, millet, quinoa, spelt, and rye

Herbs & spices
Including teas and coffee

Protein-rich foods
Including legumes (beans and pulses) and oily fish

Fruits
Mainly fresh

Fat-rich foods
Including olive oil, nuts, and seeds

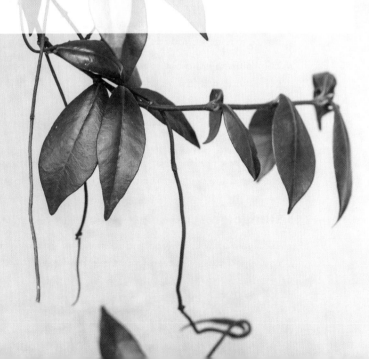

Seven Principles

1. **Mostly plants:** From fiber to prebiotics and polyphenols, there is no question that plants are our GM's favorite food.

2. **Diversity all the way:** It's all about feeding and maintaining our diversely skilled team of microbes. Remember: They all prefer different plant-based foods.

3. **Whole and natural versus refined and "perfect":** Less waste, more nutrients; it's a no-brainer.

4. **Herb and spice up your life:** There's a whole other world of flavors waiting for your taste buds (and GM) to discover.

5. **Get among legumes:** This underrated "superfood" group, loaded with prebiotics and fiber, is cost efficient, nutrient dense, and widely available.

6. **Dabble in fermented food:** It really is the ultimate way to engage with our microbial residents, not to mention the incredible flavors and textures that result.

7. **Taste, explore, pause, and enjoy:** Food is about more than just our health; it's also about community, culture, and experiences. Focusing only on the health aspect can sabotage our relationship with food, which, perhaps not surprisingly, is linked with higher rates of gut issues. Our GM can sense the unrest!

Breaking Down Barriers

When it comes to changing our eating habits, having the knowledge about what to eat is just one hurdle. So let's troubleshoot some of the other common barriers.

Access: Depending on where you live, you may be limited by the range of plant-based foods available. My motto is: Work with what you've got.

TIPS: 1) Modify recipes according to what you have—don't let a few ingredients stop you from making a dish. 2) Consider the occasional bulk buy online, particularly of dried foods such as whole grains, legumes, nuts, and seeds. 3) Try growing your own fresh herbs, spices, and sprouts (see page 293).

Time: We all have those crazy periods when we tend to push homemade meals way down our priority list. But let me challenge this way of thinking: Isn't it exactly during these periods when you need to be on top of your game? Can you really afford to get ill when you're so busy? So how do we fit it in?

TIPS:1) Frozen vegetables are underrated; they should be a staple in every busy person's freezer. 2) Meal-prep for the week ahead or set up a cooking schedule with your partner, housemates, or work colleagues. 3) Make a list of quick meals; here are some quick options that have saved me on many occasions: the Two-Minute Scramble (page 220), Thick Protein Shake (page 220), and the Creamy Pistachio and Spinach Pesto Pasta (page 249).

Cooking: I know the thought of cooking can be intimidating. But, from one cooking novice to another, you can't go wrong with most of the recipes in this book.

TIP: YouTube is a great source for quick and basic cooking tips, like how to boil the perfect egg or use a mandoline slicer.

Taste: Eating wholesome food can be terribly bland, but so can most foods if you don't dress them right.

TIP: For me, cooking is all about flaunting a food's assets; a quick dressing or fifteen minutes in the oven with some olive oil can take a food from a 5/10 to a 10/10.

Budget: Don't let your diet diversity goals stop you from buying in bulk to save.

TIP: Team up with a friend and split your purchases or freeze half the portion—most fruit and vegetables last several months in the freezer.

Plant-Based Diversity Planner

To get the most out of your diet, a little planning can go a long way. To start off with, it can be helpful to reflect on how many plant points you're currently eating on a regular basis. Over the past seven days, record the number of different plant-based foods you've eaten.

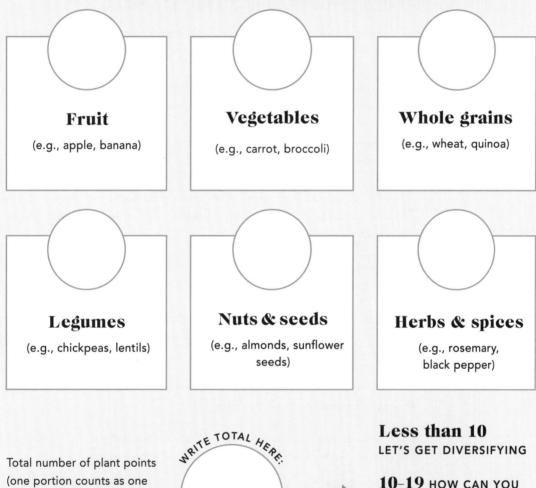

Fruit
(e.g., apple, banana)

Vegetables
(e.g., carrot, broccoli)

Whole grains
(e.g., wheat, quinoa)

Legumes
(e.g., chickpeas, lentils)

Nuts & seeds
(e.g., almonds, sunflower seeds)

Herbs & spices
(e.g., rosemary, black pepper)

Total number of plant points (one portion counts as one point; herbs and spices count as a quarter of a point):

WRITE TOTAL HERE:

Less than 10
LET'S GET DIVERSIFYING

10–19 HOW CAN YOU ADD MORE DIVERSITY?

20–29 NEARLY THERE

30+ WELL DONE!

9 Ways to Diversify Your Diet

CHECK OFF THE STRATEGIES YOU'RE GOING TO PUT INTO PRACTICE

◯ **1** Buy premixed combinations of salad and vegetables. (Instead of buying one type of salad leaf, buy a bag with grated carrot, cabbage, and sprouts, too.)

◯ **2** Experiment with grains outside your comfort zone. (Have you ever tried freekeh? If your local shop doesn't stock it, try online; it travels well.)

◯ **3** Make a grocery list before you hit the shops to avoid reverting to the same habit buys.

◯ **4** Empty a package of mixed seeds into a glass bottle and leave it on your dining table. It's a great way to remind you to sprinkle them on your meals, as you would pepper.

◯ **5** Motivation is a big part of changing habits. If competition gets you going, why not turn this into an office or family challenge?

◯ **6** Get the kids involved: Allow them to choose, buy, and even help prepare their "new" plant-based food for the week. Taking ownership is a great way to get the family on board.

◯ **7** Sometimes, inspiration is half the battle; check out page 67 for a range of plant-based foods worth trying.

◯ **8** Mix up your preparation methods. If you steamed your vegetables last night, why not add some olive oil and bake them tonight?

◯ **9** Experiment with different combinations of herbs and spices using the tips on the next page.

Herb and Spice Up Your Life

Keep a range of dried herbs and spices on your kitchen counter as a daily reminder.

Start by adding a small amount to your frying pan (two shakes) and taste as you go.

If you're just starting out in the kitchen, opt for the premixed herb and spice combinations, and just start with one per dish.

If you're only adding small amounts and tasting as you go, it's hard to go wrong, but here are some basic combos to build your confidence.

- LEGUMES: cayenne, cumin, parsley, red pepper flakes, sage, thyme

- STIR-FRY: basil, bay leaves, celery seed, cinnamon, curry, dill, fennel, garlic, ginger, oregano, parsley, red pepper flakes, rosemary, smoked paprika, thyme

- SALAD DRESSINGS: basil, celery seed, chives, dill, fennel, horseradish, mint, mustard, oregano, paprika, parsley, pepper, saffron

- BREADS & CRACKERS: basil, caraway, cardamom, coriander, cumin, dill, orange peel, oregano, poppy seeds, rosemary, saffron, sage, thyme

- FRUITS: allspice, anise, cardamom, cinnamon, cloves, coriander, ginger, mint

- DESSERTS: allspice, anise, cardamom, cinnamon, cloves, fennel, ginger, lemon peel, mace, nutmeg, mint, orange peel, rosemary

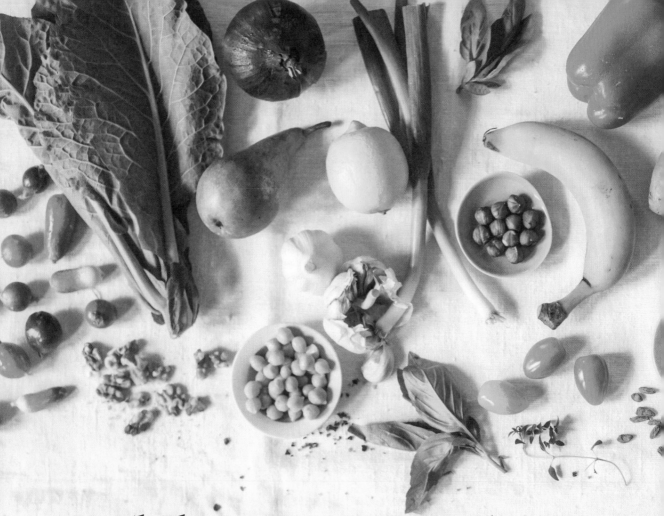

Month Planner

When it comes to dietary changes, for most people, slow and steady wins the race. With this in mind, to achieve your diversity target, I find that starting by adding just one or two new varieties each week is the best way to manage and achieve your goal.

WEEK 1: PLANT-BASED FOODS TO TRY	WEEK 2: PLANT-BASED FOODS TO TRY

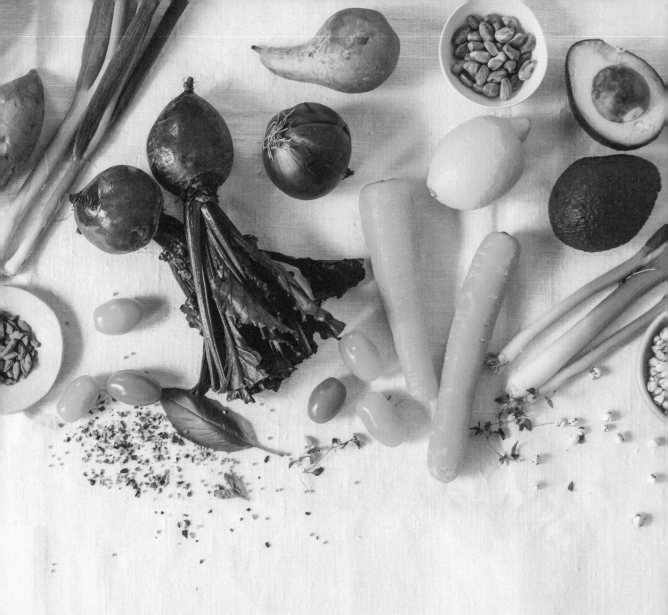

WEEK 3: PLANT-BASED FOODS TO TRY

WEEK 4: PLANT-BASED FOODS TO TRY

CHAPTER 4

Common Complaints

Common Complaints and How to Manage Them

Whether it's an occasional inconvenience or a debilitating daily occurrence, no one should have to put up with ongoing gut distress. Unfortunately, many do—in fact, a national survey found that nearly two out of three people in the US are burdened by gut symptoms.[27] So, what do most do when faced with this type of burden? Check in with Dr. Google, of course! Whether it's the convenience factor, the potential for embarrassment, or the intimidating thought of a complex array of investigations and medication, many avoid heading to their doctor—I totally get it.

But you don't need to turn to the internet anymore. Instead, I want to welcome you to this safe, evidence-based space where we'll address the most common gut complaints and discuss practical strategies to help you deal with them. This chapter is certainly not designed to replace your doctor or dietitian, but it will point you in the right direction of what you need to do to shake those bothersome symptoms, from simple home solutions to knowing when to visit relevant healthcare professionals.

The strategies covered in this chapter are grounded in evidence from quality trials, observational studies, expert consensus, and sound understanding of how the gut works. Throughout this chapter, I've prioritized the top-quality trials when providing advice. Where there aren't any, I've suggested strategies that, although they don't have a wealth of research to back them up, are safe and have worked for many of my patients. There's that motto again: Let's work with what we've got!

> ✋ **Caution:** *If you have a history of disordered eating, please seek support from a dietitian before considering any of the dietary strategies to come. Despite good intentions, focusing on specific aspects of food can trigger negative thoughts and relapse.*

Before you start testing out the strategies outlined in this chapter it's a good idea to complete the Gut Feelings assessment on page 21, so that you have an objective record of your symptoms. For each of the diet strategies, unless otherwise specified, I recommend that you follow the advice for around four weeks. At the end of the four weeks, repeat the same symptom assessment. This will give you an objective idea about whether the intervention worked for you. If there's no improvement, go back to your usual diet and, after a few weeks, reassess your symptoms and move on to the next strategy. Reassessing the changes in your symptoms once you've returned to your normal diet, although it sounds a bit cumbersome, is actually rather valuable in confirming whether it has worked. If your symptoms do improve, this chapter will also look at how to embed the changes into your everyday life without them becoming a burden or placing you at risk of nutritional inadequacies.

Assessment: GUT-BRAIN ASSESSMENT

I love this tool, because it helps gauge whether centrally targeted strategies, that is, those that target the messages traveling from your brain to your gut (the gut-brain axis), are going to be important in your management plan. Only complete this assessment if you selected at least three moderate gut symptoms in the Gut Feelings assessment on page 21.

The following statements describe how some of us respond to symptoms in our gut. Answer how strongly you agree or disagree with each of these statements, as they relate to you. These answers are to help personalize the way you manage your gut symptoms, so try to answer as accurately and honestly as you can.

	Strongly agree	Moderately agree	Slightly agree	Slightly disagree	Moderately disagree	Strongly disagree
1. I worry that whenever I eat during the day, bloating and distension in my belly will get worse.	1	2	3	4	5	6
2. I get anxious when I go to a new restaurant.	1	2	3	4	5	6
3. I often worry about problems in my belly.	1	2	3	4	5	6
4. I have a difficult time enjoying myself because I cannot get my mind off of discomfort in my belly.	1	2	3	4	5	6
5. I often fear that I won't be able to have a normal bowel movement.	1	2	3	4	5	6
6. Because of fear of developing abdominal discomfort, I rarely try new foods.	1	2	3	4	5	6
7. No matter what I eat, I will probably feel uncomfortable.	1	2	3	4	5	6
8. As soon as I feel abdominal discomfort, I begin to worry and feel anxious.	1	2	3	4	5	6
9. When I enter a place I haven't been before, one of the first things I do is to look for a bathroom.	1	2	3	4	5	6
10. I am constantly aware of the feelings I have in my belly.						

(assessment continues)

	Strongly agree	Moderately agree	Slightly agree	Slightly disagree	Moderately disagree	Strongly disagree
11. I often feel that discomfort in my belly could be a sign of a serious illness.	1	2	3	4	5	6
12. As soon as I wake, I worry that I will have discomfort in my belly during the day.	1	2	3	4	5	6
13. When I feel discomfort in my belly, it frightens me.	1	2	3	4	5	6
14. In stressful situations, my belly bothers me a lot.	1	2	3	4	5	6
15. I constantly think about what is happening inside my belly.	1	2	3	4	5	6

Source: Alimentary Pharmacology & Therapeutics[28]

SCORE INTERPRETATION

Altered central stress response   Normal central stress response

15 points   ━━━━━━━━━━▶   90 points

If your score is toward the lower end of this scale, psychological factors, including certain forms of stress, as well as gut-specific anxiety, are likely to be playing a role in maintaining and even exacerbating your gut symptoms. This is not to say that your symptoms are all in your head (I hate it when I hear that, because it shows the depth of people's misunderstanding); what it is suggesting is that the signals going from your brain to your gut are out of whack, triggering your symptoms, at least to some degree. With this in mind, if your score is below 60, I recommend that you also include strategies that target your central nervous system (your brain) in your Gut-Health Action Plan on page 210. We'll discuss this in chapter 6.

Constipation

The word *constipation* can mean different things to different people. For some, it's all about how often they poop, whereas others associate it with straining, not emptying their bowels completely, or the consistency of their poop. These are all valid descriptions. There are three main subtypes of constipation:

1. SLOW TRANSIT CONSTIPATION: This is when poop takes a long time to move through the large intestine. This slow movement means there is more time for water to be absorbed, leaving you with a hard, dry poop.

2. EVACUATION DISORDER: Everything moves at a normal speed through the large intestine, but something's not quite right with the final "push," resulting in constipation. This might be due to poorly orchestrated bowel movements involved in pooping, including the intestine, anal sphincter, and pelvic-floor muscles. This means that things are moving, but not in a coordinated fashion (kind of like me on the dance floor). This can result from problematic childhood toilet habits or be due to physical or structural problems, such as a collapse of the intestinal wall into the vagina (known as a rectocele).

Common Symptoms of a Rectocele

- *Feeling like there is something coming down into your vagina (it may feel like you're sitting on a small ball)*
- *Feeling or seeing a bulge in or coming out of your vagina*
- *Pressure or pain in your bottom*
- *Discomfort or numbness during sex*

3. CONSTIPATION-PREDOMINANT IRRITABLE BOWEL SYNDROME (IBS): There are four types of IBS, and one is dominated by constipation. For some, managing constipation can improve other symptoms of IBS, including gut pain and bloating. Trying the strategies in this chapter can be a useful first step.

Potential Causes of Constipation

LOW LEVELS OF ACTIVITY: Decreased stimulation of gut muscles.

STRESS, ANXIETY, OR DEPRESSION: Altered communication via the gut-brain axis.

PREGNANCY: Both hormonal changes and the physical compression of the uterus on the intestine.

CHANGES IN ROUTINE: Our bowels are creatures of habit, and changing your eating and sleeping times can confuse them.

IGNORING THE URGE TO GO: This allows more time for water to be absorbed, resulting in a hard and dry poop, which is difficult for your gut to push out.

NOT EATING ENOUGH WHOLE-GRAIN FIBER: Whole-grain fiber can help add bulk to poop, giving your gut muscles more to work with.

CHILDHOOD TOILETING: Feeling pressured or being regularly interrupted can lead to the development of poor pooping habits.

HISTORY OF PHYSICAL OR PSYCHOLOGICAL ABUSE: Trauma can affect the function of muscles involved in pooping via the gut-brain axis.

MEDICATION OR SUPPLEMENTS: Different types can affect the bowels, by directly interfering with the gut muscle movements or increasing fluid absorption.

Taking Action

Managing constipation isn't one-size-fits-all. To help find the strategies that are right for you, I've developed this decision flowchart. It's as easy as following the arrows and answering the questions as you go. There are three broad areas: diet, physical activity, and toilet habits.

For best results, try one strategy from each area.

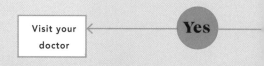

Visit your doctor ◄── **Yes**

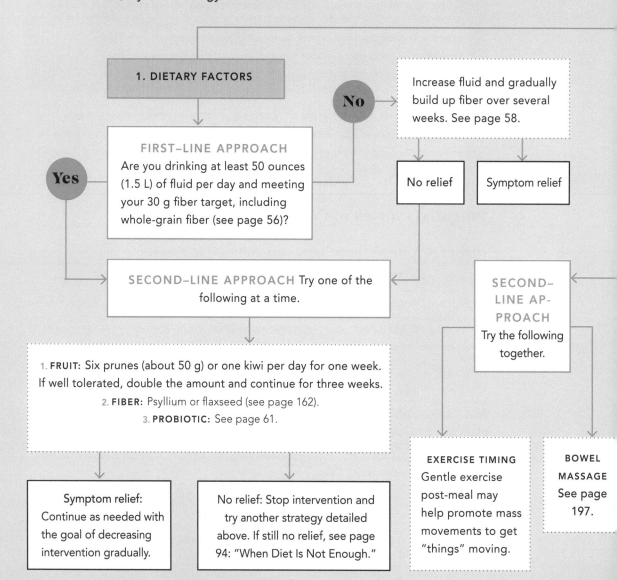

1. DIETARY FACTORS

No → Increase fluid and gradually build up fiber over several weeks. See page 58.

↓ No relief   Symptom relief

FIRST–LINE APPROACH
Are you drinking at least 50 ounces (1.5 L) of fluid per day and meeting your 30 g fiber target, including whole-grain fiber (see page 56)?

Yes

SECOND–LINE APPROACH Try one of the following at a time.

SECOND–LINE APPROACH
Try the following together.

1. **FRUIT:** Six prunes (about 50 g) or one kiwi per day for one week. If well tolerated, double the amount and continue for three weeks.
2. **FIBER:** Psyllium or flaxseed (see page 162).
3. **PROBIOTIC:** See page 61.

Symptom relief: Continue as needed with the goal of decreasing intervention gradually.

No relief: Stop intervention and try another strategy detailed above. If still no relief, see page 94: "When Diet Is Not Enough."

EXERCISE TIMING Gentle exercise post-meal may help promote mass movements to get "things" moving.

BOWEL MASSAGE See page 197.

Constipation

DO YOU HAVE ANY ALARM FEATURES?
SEE PAGE 89

No → LIFESTYLE CHANGES

2. PHYSICAL ACTIVITY

3. TOILET HABITS

Yes

FIRST–LINE APPROACH
Do you exercise at least three times per week (for at least 30 minutes) to a level where you'd become short of breath if you tried to sing?

No

Whether it's power walking with a friend, going dancing, or joining a sports team, regularly moving your body can make a big difference.

ROUTINE
1. Give yourself five to ten minutes to sit and relax on the toilet; even if you don't poop, make this part of your daily routine. Don't pressure or strain your bowels, either; they'll go when they feel comfortable. You may find that listening to music or a mindfulness app can help relax you.

2. Aim to sit on the toilet at the same time each day. The mass movement in the morning increases post-meal and after coffee, so try to maximize your chances by dedicating time then.

POSITIONING AND TECHNIQUE
1. Check in with your pooping position on page 195.

2. Train your pooping muscles on page 196.

LISTEN TO YOUR BODY
When you get the urge, go! Withholding can cause constipation.

When Diet Is Not Enough

Like each of us, our bowels are unique and have their own "personalities." Some are laid-back and easygoing, while others can be a little more uptight and reliant on routine. This explains why there is no single strategy or medication that suits all. Take two of my patients: thirty-nine-year-old Sally and twenty-seven-year-old Jenny. They both presented with near-identical gut symptoms but, as I got to know more about each of them, it became strikingly clear how different their bowel personalities were. Sally's bowels were a happy-go-lucky type that just needed more fiber to give the muscles something to work with. Psyllium worked really well, and we followed by increasing the whole grains in her diet, for long-term maintenance. Then there was Jenny. At face value, it seemed Jenny's bowels were plain old stubborn. Jenny had a high-fiber diet, drank plenty of water, and exercised five days a week. When she came to me, she was juggling different laxatives and struggling to get the balance right in terms of dose and frequency, having had many "close calls" at work. We sat together and got to know her bowels. We learned that they were not stubborn but shy: They didn't like opening anywhere but in the comfort of her own home. In fact, when Jenny was housesitting with her boyfriend, her bowels were so self-conscious that they didn't open all week. For Jenny's bowels, it was all about creating a feeling of comfort and safety. We started off by establishing a relaxing morning bowel routine, while slowly cutting down the laxatives. Jenny also started using the Poop-Pourri (see recipe on opposite page) when she needed to go outside of her comfort zone. Within three weeks, Jenny was laxative-free and not only had her bowel confidence been boosted, but her anxiety had also reduced, with no more worrying about laxative-related incidents.

Laxatives

In cases where things are pretty "backed up," sometimes you need an extra push to get things moving, at least initially. It's always best to discuss with your pharmacist before starting, as laxatives can make some conditions worse. There are also laxatives that your doctor can prescribe if over-the-counter laxatives are not effective. If you find yourself depending on laxatives for more than a week, visit your doctor to discuss different options.

Poop-Pourri

Now, don't laugh: This really will revolutionize your bathroom experience. Not only does it smell so much more natural and subtler than traditional toilet sprays, but it's also a tenth of the price, and so much more efficient at getting the "job" done. The role of this concoction is not to mask the smell in the air that escapes the toilet bowl but rather to trap the smell inside the toilet bowl. I know it sounds a little too good to be true, but it's no marketing scam; it's just based on simple science! Spray this directly into the bowl before you go. The oily mix forms a thin film across the water in the toilet, so when you go, it traps the smell (which is just a mix of gases produced by our GM) under the film. When you flush the toilet, the smell is gone—like magic. It also makes a very memorable (and affordable) present for your friends and family. You can also place the bottle in your bathroom with written instructions for your guests on how to use it.

You will need one 2-ounce (60 ml) glass spray bottle (plastic is OK for short-term use)

10 to 15 drops essential oils of choice (I like peppermint or a combo of lavender and vanilla)
1 tablespoon rubbing alcohol (or 2 tablespoons vodka)
1 pea-sized drop body wash or liquid soap (this helps combine the oil and water)
Distilled water (tap water is fine if you use within one month)

1. Pour the essential oils and the alcohol into your spray bottle and shake well.

2. Add the body wash or liquid soap, then fill the bottle up to the neck with water. Shake well.

3. Place in your bathroom. To use, shake well, then spray four times into the toilet bowl, pre-poop.

Bloating

Bloating is one of the most common gut symptoms people report and can be rather distressing, especially when the cause is unexplained.

Bloating is the feeling of increased pressure in your intestine that may be accompanied by visible protrusion (aka a "food baby"). The causes and mechanics of bloating are complex. The built-up pressure can result from the sheer volume of food or fluid you've consumed or from gas produced by our gut microbiota (GM) when it's fed large amounts of fermentable carbohydrates, including some types of fiber. This increase in gut content essentially stretches the intestine, giving you the sensation of bloating.

But why do some people experience bloating and others don't, even when they eat and drink the same type and amount of food? There are many reasons, but one of the most common is the sensitivity of your intestine. A heightened sensitivity, known as visceral hypersensitivity, is particularly common in people with functional gut disorders like IBS. Visceral hypersensitivity has been demonstrated in studies that use MRI (scans that can measure gas inside your intestines). What they have shown is that, despite the same amount of gas present in the intestines, people with IBS, or other functional gut disorders, are more likely to feel bloated than those without them.

Susceptibility to bloating can also depend on the balance between how much gas your unique GM produces and how efficient your body is at absorbing it. The transport of gas through the intestine can also be an issue for some, resulting in trapped gas. Many of the strategies discussed below, such as gentle stretching, abdominal massage, and heat packs, can help release trapped gas.

In a subset of people with functional gut disorders, bloating can also be exaggerated by an inappropriate movement of the diaphragm (the dome-shaped sheet of muscle that helps us breathe) and the belly. This results in belly protrusion, which people frequently describe as making them look several months pregnant, even though they're not. It's similar to when you take a big breath into your belly, pushing it out, except it happens unconsciously. Unlike standard bloating, this has nothing to do with what's in your intestine per se; instead, it's considered a reflex related to tummy pain or discomfort whereby the gut triggers the brain via the gut-brain axis and, in an attempt to relieve the gut distress, the brain contracts the diaphragm and relaxes the tummy muscles. The fix? Once the trigger of the tummy pain or discomfort is managed (whether it's IBS, constipation, or another cause), the belly protrusion also typically resolves. In my clinic, I've also found that spending five minutes doing some diaphragmatic breathing each day for at least eight weeks can help you become more aware of when this reflex is triggered; in turn, this can help you to consciously release the over-contracted diaphragm (see page 184).

There are two main types of bloating: continuous and intermittent. Continuous bloating is always present, with no daily fluctuations or association with what you eat. This could be related to the reflex discussed above, but it may also be a sign that something more troublesome is going on, so it's best to visit your doctor to be safe. Intermittent bloating is more common, and often people report their symptoms are worse toward the end of the day or after a meal. This type is most often managed through diet and lifestyle strategies.

It's important to be aware that occasional bloating is normal, particularly if we've had a heavy meal or eaten extra fiber. In fact, a bit of bloating after a high-fiber meal is a good thing. It's a sign of a well-fed GM that's doing its job.

Despite the complexity of the causes of bloating, it can be reduced in many cases, or even eliminated, with simple changes to diet and lifestyle. These self-management strategies can be broken down into two stages in order of difficulty, starting with low-burden strategies and working up. As always, it's up to you which stage you start at, but I recommend starting with the "low-hanging fruit," so to speak, and working through the more time-consuming strategies only if needed. For many people, first-line strategies are enough.

What Are "Functional" Gut Disorders?

This is a category of conditions that include IBS, where the structure of the gut is normal but the function isn't. Somewhat like a model home, everything looks OK but, on closer inspection, the plumbing and electricity don't actually work. If it turns out that this applies to your gut, don't panic, as such disorders really are very common (we'll assess this on page 145).

1. First-Line Strategies

Diet

AVOID LARGE MEALS. Split food intake into smaller portions, eating four or five meals spread across the day.

TAKE TIME TO CHEW YOUR FOOD WELL, aiming for between ten and twenty chews per mouthful. It can also help to get into the habit of putting down your knife and fork after each mouthful to remind yourself to take time to chew.

Although the evidence is limited, AVOID SWALLOWING EXCESS AIR from carbonated drinks, drinking through a straw, and chewing gum.

AVOID ADDED POLYOLS that are commonly found in sugar-free foods and chewing gum, such as mannitol, maltitol, sorbitol, xylitol, and isomalt.

ARE YOU OVERDOING IT ON FERMENTED FOODS (E.G., KEFIR, SAUERKRAUT)? Halve your portions for two weeks and reassess. If your symptoms improve, continue with smaller portions and look to gradually increase over time, if appropriate.

KEEP TO NO MORE THAN ONE PIECE OF FRUIT PER SITTING (about 3 ounces/80 g fresh or 1 ounce/30 g dried), with up to three servings per day.

AVOID SMOOTHIES AND JUICES. Opt for whole foods instead.

Lifestyle

AVOID WEARING TIGHT CLOTHES. I know this sounds a little odd, but "tight pants syndrome" is actually a thing! It was first described in a medical journal back in 1993.[29]

GENTLE EXERCISE AND STRETCHING CAN HELP DIFFUSE TRAPPED GAS. Check out the yoga flow on page 183.

BETTER OUT THAN IN. Go for a walk outside and "deflate."

TRY PEPPERMINT OIL CAPSULES. Peppermint oil has been shown to relax your gut muscles and therefore may help relieve bloating triggered by trapped gas. The evidence for peppermint oil and bloating is based on results in people with IBS. See page 163.

TRY USING A HEAT PACK. Placing a heat pack (or a warm damp towel) on your belly can help loosen up the gut muscles, which may relieve trapped gas. This also recruits more blood flow to the area, which may settle overactive gut muscles.

It's up to you whether you want to try one strategy at a time or choose a few. If symptoms do improve with multiple strategies, you may like to reintroduce each strategy one by one. This will help you to assess which are most beneficial so you're not burdened with too many changes in the long term. If you don't get symptom relief from the first-line strategies, move on to the second-line strategies.

Remember: *Include chosen strategies in your Gut-Health Action Plan on page 210.*

2. Second-Line Strategies

Diet

CHECK FOR FOOD INTOLERANCES—see chapter 5.

HALVE YOUR PORTIONS OF KEY HIGHER-FODMAP FOODS from the table on page 159 for two weeks. If symptoms improve, reintroduce as per Stage 2: Reintroduction on page 160. If symptoms only slightly improve, you may like to consider the full FODMAP-Lite approach on pages 160 and 161.

Additional Therapies

CONSIDER STRATEGIES THAT TARGET THE GUT-BRAIN AXIS in chapter 7.

DISCUSS FURTHER INVESTIGATIONS WITH YOUR DOCTOR, including small intestinal bacterial overgrowth (SIBO; page 164) and celiac disease (page 115).

Bloating can also be a side effect of constipation and diarrhea. If you suffer from either, make sure you check out those symptom-specific strategies, too (pages 92, 93, and 101).

Although we tend to blame bloating all on diet, I find this is rarely the case. This was certainly true for one of my patients, twenty-nine-year-old Catherine. Catherine was an ex-gymnast who, although professionally retired, was still training most days. She struggled with bloating, alongside what she called "moody bowels" for several years (the type that switch from hard to loose from one week to the next). But it wasn't until she was out at a dinner party and received the attempted compliment, "You look fantastic, how far along are you?" that Catherine was driven to take action. In my clinic, Catherine told me the details of her diet and lifestyle and opened up about her history of anorexia. Although she had recovered from her eating disorder, it was apparent that her bowels were still in the process of repairing themselves. I explained to Catherine that, just like our arm and leg muscles, we can also lose gut muscle when severely malnourished, as in the case of anorexia. As a result, the way in which the nerves and gut muscles communicate can become impaired, resulting in these bothersome gut symptoms. I also reinforced the message that, although, for most, this nerve-muscle communication tends to resolve with time, it was important to be realistic with her expectations and to acknowledge that things can take a little longer for some than it might for others. Catherine had also recognized that the more frustrated she got with her bloating, the worse it seemed to get.

How did we approach it? Slowly and gently was the key. We identified several lifestyle factors, including stress (particularly food-related fears from previous learned behaviors) and wearing tight gym gear all day. In terms of diet, Catherine was taking large amounts of a prebiotic supplement (which she had read was good for her gut), so we cut that out and focused on getting all her required nutrition from five smaller meals spread across the day. We didn't restrict any foods but instead broadened her diet in line with the Gut Health on a Plate principles from chapter 3. Over the following six months, Catherine managed to get on top of her gut symptoms and also noticed an improvement in her mental health. In fact, when I asked her how she was feeling, she remarked, after a moment of thought, "You know what, I feel like a new woman."

Diarrhea

Loose or watery poop occurs when there is either too much fluid secreted into the intestine or not enough fluid reabsorbed into your body. Here's a fun fact for you: On average, a massive 300 ounces (9 L) of fluid enters the small intestine each day, mainly from body secretions, of which 90 percent is normally reabsorbed.

When thinking about how to manage diarrhea, consider whether it's an acute (short-term) or chronic (longer-term) issue. Diarrhea can also come with other symptoms, such as urgency (not being able to hold it back). If you're nodding right now, rest assured, there are several strategies to help you get on top of it.

Acute Diarrhea

Acute diarrhea is often caused by the invasion of unfriendly microbes into the intestine. This may last from a few days to several weeks, and includes traveler's diarrhea, viral gastroenteritis ("enteritis" meaning inflammation of the small intestine), and food poisoning. This type of diarrhea can also occur when you start a new medication, including antibiotics. Acute diarrhea is best managed by your doctor, who can assess whether medication is needed.

- **TRAVELER'S DIARRHEA:** This is the most common illness in travelers visiting developing countries, with reports suggesting that it affects between 20 and 50 percent of travelers.[30] Although the diarrhea is usually mild and can be self-managed, as many as 10 percent of sufferers may go on to develop what is called post-infectious IBS (discussed in chapter 6). It's best to see your doctor before taking any antidiarrheal medication for acute diarrhea, as it may prolong an infection by trapping the culprit in the intestine.

- **ANTIBIOTIC-ASSOCIATED DIARRHEA:** Although antibiotics are crucial in fighting off some bacterial infections, they can also disrupt your GM, which can result in diarrhea. As many as 30 percent of people are said to experience loose poops when taking antibiotics. To combat this, taking a specific probiotic during your antibiotic therapy and continuing for a week post-antibiotics has been shown to significantly decrease your risk of AAD.

Chronic Diarrhea

Chronic diarrhea is a nonspecific symptom that can occur because of a functional gut disorder or a more sinister problem. If it's accompanied by any of the alarm features on page 89, visit your doctor as a first step.

Treatment of chronic diarrhea is best achieved by managing the underlying cause. This might mean identifying a food intolerance or identifying and medically managing the disease (e.g., IBD). There are also several strategies that can help manage symptoms, particularly if symptoms persist following medical management.

Diet Strategies

EAT SMALLER, MORE FREQUENT MEALS. A good rule of thumb is to divide your current meals into five or six smaller meals across the day, meaning you don't change the total amount you eat, just your eating pattern.

LIMIT FOODS AND FLUIDS THAT MAY STIMULATE THE COLON, such as chile peppers, high-fat meals, coffee, and alcohol.

LIMIT KEY SOURCES OF FERMENTABLE CARBOHYDRATES (higher-FODMAP foods; see page 159) for two weeks, followed by reintroduction (page 160).

If diarrhea is severe, ENSURE ADEQUATE HYDRATION WITH ELECTROLYTE SOLUTION, such as Pedialyte. This is needed when fluid is passing "straight through."

CONSIDER PSYLLIUM HUSK. This is a water-loving fiber that can help thicken your poop. Check out page 162 for more details.

Lifestyle Strategies

AVOID NICOTINE, which may stimulate gut movements.

If suffering from urgency or pooping mishaps, DAILY PELVIC FLOOR EXERCISES can help (see page 196).

If psyllium doesn't help, DISCUSS THE USE OF AN ANTIDIARRHEAL WITH YOUR DOCTOR. This will slow down gut movement, allowing more time for gut fluid to be reabsorbed. First-line antimotility medications include loperamide (Imodium).

NOTE: Antimotility medications may be less well tolerated in diarrhea-predominant IBS.

Flatulence

Breaking wind, cutting the cheese, letting one rip—however you refer to it, flatulence is a normal, healthy phenomenon. The average person meeting their daily 30 grams of fiber passes flatus (wind) between ten and twenty times a day. This is a sign of a well-fed GM, but if flatulence becomes persistently excessive or the smell is a cause for a building evacuation and it interferes with your work or social life, keep reading. Gas in our intestines comes from two main sources: from the air we breathe in and as the by-product of GM fermentation in the large intestine (from our GM digesting our food leftovers). When it comes to flatulence, the gas produced by our GM is the most relevant source. This explains why around 70 percent of total gas in the intestine in healthy people is found in the large intestine.

When looking to manage flatulence, as daft as it may sound, it's worth considering which aspect bothers you. Typically, if you're passing wind less than twenty times a day, it's more likely other factors that are bothering you. Is it the odor, the inability to hold it back, or the soiling of underwear that can sometimes occur? Although each can be socially embarrassing, if you identify the problem, it will help inform the most effective management strategies to solve it.

Excess Gas

Excess gas is typically the result of excess GM fermentation, which may mean that you've overfed your GM. There are many causes for excess GM fermentation:

EXCESS FOOD RESIDUE: Our GM engages in a feeding frenzy if too much food gets to the large intestine. This can occur in several scenarios, like when food travels too fast through the small intestine (diarrhea); if you're unable to digest specific food components (food intolerance); or if you have a really high-fiber diet or rapidly increase the amount of fiber you eat.

CONSTIPATION: If things travel extra slowly through the large intestine, the GM gets more time to ferment the leftover food bits that would otherwise have exited into the toilet bowl.

SMALL INTESTINE BACTERIAL OVERGROWTH (SIBO): When a considerable number of bacteria travel up from the large intestine into the small intestine, these bacteria suddenly have access to all that lovely food that they didn't have access to in the large intestine (see page 164 for more on SIBO).

Odor

Interestingly, more than 99 percent of the gas produced by our GM, including hydrogen, methane, and carbon dioxide, is odorless. So where's the smell coming from? That distinct whiff of rotten egg is caused by bacteria breaking down sulfur-containing compounds in our diet. This produces trace amounts of sulfur-containing gases such as hydrogen sulfide. Food and/or drinks high in sulfur-containing compounds include those high in specific amino acids (the building blocks of protein: cysteine, methionine, and taurine). These include protein supplements, meat, chicken, eggs, and so on. Sulfur-containing compounds are also found in cruciferous vegetables (e.g., broccoli, cauliflower, cabbage, kale, brussels sprouts, and turnips), allium vegetables (e.g., garlic, onion, leeks, and chives), and additives (e.g., some beer and wine).

But before you go cutting out these types of vegetables, it's worth noting that many of their sulfur-containing compounds are known to have a range of health benefits, and their rotten-egg potential is also much lower than high-protein foods such as protein supplements (both whey- and plant-based). Therefore, targeting the excess protein intake is a better place to start. Interestingly, in contrast to traditional thinking, research from Dr. CK Yao and colleagues suggests that increasing fiber, rather than restricting it, may in fact help manage pungent flatulence.[31] How? By increasing the availability of dietary fiber, our GM is kept busy feeding on that and is less likely to ferment the sulfur-containing amino acids found in high-protein foods.

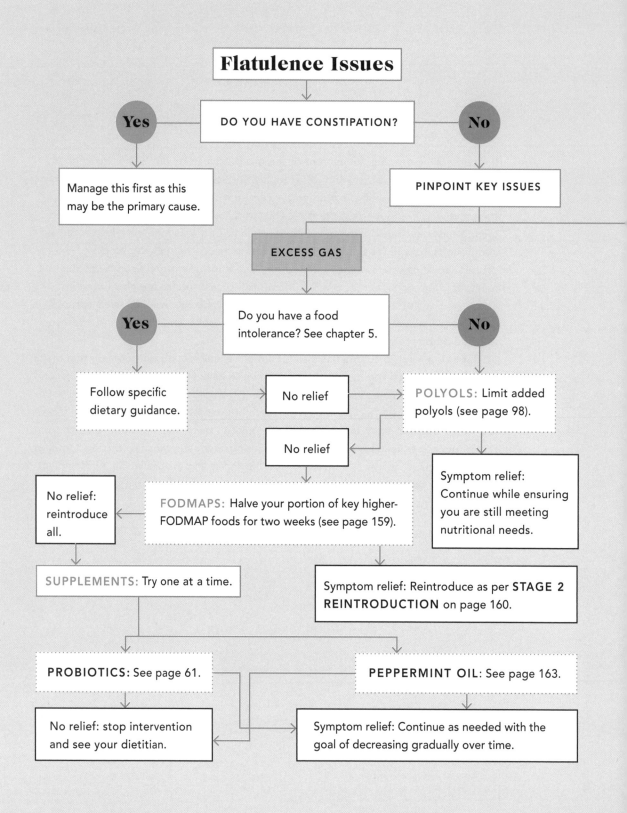

Flatulence Issues

Yes ← **DO YOU HAVE CONSTIPATION?** → **No**

Manage this first as this may be the primary cause.

PINPOINT KEY ISSUES

EXCESS GAS

Yes ← Do you have a food intolerance? See chapter 5. → **No**

Follow specific dietary guidance. → No relief → POLYOLS: Limit added polyols (see page 98).

No relief ←

Symptom relief: Continue while ensuring you are still meeting nutritional needs.

No relief: reintroduce all. ← FODMAPS: Halve your portion of key higher-FODMAP foods for two weeks (see page 159).

SUPPLEMENTS: Try one at a time.

Symptom relief: Reintroduce as per **STAGE 2 REINTRODUCTION** on page 160.

PROBIOTICS: See page 61.   PEPPERMINT OIL: See page 163.

No relief: stop intervention and see your dietitian.

Symptom relief: Continue as needed with the goal of decreasing gradually over time.

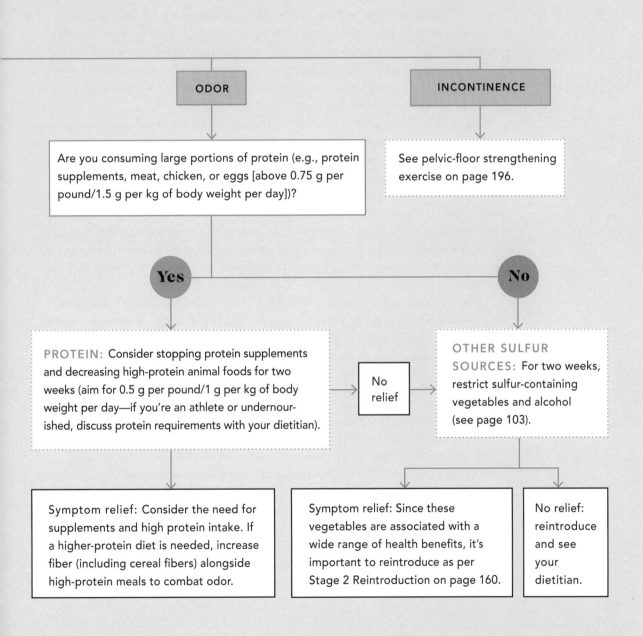

ODOR

INCONTINENCE

Are you consuming large portions of protein (e.g., protein supplements, meat, chicken, or eggs [above 0.75 g per pound/1.5 g per kg of body weight per day])?

See pelvic-floor strengthening exercise on page 196.

Yes

No

PROTEIN: Consider stopping protein supplements and decreasing high-protein animal foods for two weeks (aim for 0.5 g per pound/1 g per kg of body weight per day—if you're an athlete or undernourished, discuss protein requirements with your dietitian).

No relief

OTHER SULFUR SOURCES: For two weeks, restrict sulfur-containing vegetables and alcohol (see page 103).

Symptom relief: Consider the need for supplements and high protein intake. If a higher-protein diet is needed, increase fiber (including cereal fibers) alongside high-protein meals to combat odor.

Symptom relief: Since these vegetables are associated with a wide range of health benefits, it's important to reintroduce as per Stage 2 Reintroduction on page 160.

No relief: reintroduce and see your dietitian.

Heartburn and Acid Reflux

Despite its misleading name and the location of the symptoms, heartburn has nothing to do with the heart—it's all about your esophagus (food pipe). Heartburn is a common symptom of reflux, where acid travels in the wrong direction, up from your stomach and into your esophagus via the esophageal sphincter (we covered this in chapter 1). Unlike your stomach, your esophagus isn't built for harsh acid, so the acid triggers a nasty burning sensation in the chest: heartburn.

Most people will experience heartburn if they overfill their stomach and thus create an unequal pressure between the stomach and esophagus. When this pressure imbalance reaches a certain level, it essentially lifts the sphincter "trapdoor" and allows acid to flow upward into the esophagus. If, however, you're experiencing heartburn and/or reflux regularly (at least twice a week), and it's not related to overeating, you may have what's called gastroesophageal reflux disease (GERD). GERD is a common condition, affecting more than 10 percent of adults in the US.[32] Although some people are genetically more susceptible to reflux, and others have a physical cause such as a hiatus hernia, there are several key diet and lifestyle factors (outlined on page 108) that can decrease your risk of GERD.

Not all heartburn occurs because of acid reflux. This explains why, for some people, acid reflux medications (even the strong ones) provide no relief. This type of heartburn, where there is no clinical explanation or abnormal test, is termed "functional heartburn" (yes, that word *functional* again). Like the other functional gut disorders, a sensitive intestine, related to the dysfunction between the gut and the brain, is thought to play a role.

This was the case with one of my patients, fifty-two-year-old Tom. Tom had been bothered by symptoms of heartburn on and off for ten years, although, over the last year, his symptoms had become progressively worse. Tom's doctor had prescribed him a proton-pump inhibitor (which works to lower stomach acid production). After several months and no benefit (despite increasing the dose), he was referred for an endoscopy (where they pass a camera down the esophagus) to take a look at what was going on. He also had other tests to find out how the esophagus was moving and how much acid was entering. All the tests came back normal. At this stage, Tom was at a bit of a loss as to what was going on, so decided to come and see me. He explained that he had tried all the standard diet strategies, but none of them had worked. Appreciating the functional nature of Tom's symptoms, we went into detail about not only Tom's diet but also other lifestyle factors, including sleep, stress, hobbies, and so on. He also opened up about his recent marriage breakdown, which was causing him a lot of stress.

We decided not to change Tom's diet (he felt this stressed him out more) and started with some basic daily mindfulness and sleep strategies (see chapter 7). I reinforced to Tom that to see the benefit he had to really commit to these daily strategies. To help with this, we went through a number of habit-forming tips (see page 206). Eight weeks later, Tom returned, his stress down and his sleep quality up. The severity of his heartburn had also lessened, although he was still feeling it most days. Having experienced some benefit, Tom was keen to take the next step and readdress some of those diet strategies, including reducing his alcohol intake and the size of his evening meal—both of which he'd previously tried, with only limited success. Four weeks later, Tom emailed me to express his gratitude and to say that he didn't need another appointment, as he had his symptoms under control.

So, what is the evidence behind diet and lifestyle strategies for managing heartburn and reflux? I'll be frank with you: It is minimal in terms of good-quality trials. But there are observational studies, and consensus from leading experts, that support trying these strategies before opting for medication. If there is a part of you that's tempted to skip these strategies and just go straight for the meds—because, let's face it, they can be easier to implement—keep in mind that some reflux medications may affect your GM. Of course, if you need medication, you need it—it's all about weighing up the pros and cons. For those tempted to just put up with the symptoms, it's important to be aware that chronic reflux is not only burdensome for you in terms of the discomfort but can also increase your risk of diseases such as esophageal cancer—so whichever pathway you decide to take, getting on top of it is really important.

Diet Strategies: Short Term

AVOID LARGE MEALS. Split food intake into smaller portions, eating five or six meals across the day.

ALLOW AT LEAST THREE HOURS between your last meal of the day and bedtime.

COMPLETE A SEVEN-DAY FOOD AND SYMPTOM DIARY (see My Gut Diary, page 128) and look for any patterns between foods, lifestyle factors, and your symptoms. Although evidence is limited, commonly reported diet triggers include high-fat meals, (e.g., deep-fried foods and pastries; switch to grilled and whole-grain options), carbonated beverages, citrus fruits and juices (try herbal teas instead), tomatoes, spicy foods (switch to another flavorful herb, like smoked paprika or turmeric), chocolate, caffeine (opt for decaffeinated drinks), and alcohol.

Diet Strategies: Long Term

KEEP YOUR WEIGHT IN CHECK, as being overweight is linked with a higher risk of reflux. This is because the extra weight increases the pressure placed on your esophageal sphincter.

CONSTIPATION AND BLOATING MAY ALSO WORSEN REFLUX, so ensure these are well managed.

Alarm Features

If you have any of the red flags below, don't hold off. Discuss with your doctor right away.

- *Difficulty swallowing*
- *Any lumps or tenderness in your throat or belly*
- *Family history of either esophageal or stomach cancer*

Lifestyle Strategies

DE-STRESS WITH BREATHING EXERCISES (SEE PAGE 184). It all comes back to the gut-brain axis, where mental stress can trigger physical stress along your intestine.

AVOID TIGHT CLOTHING, like high-waisted jeans or tight bras.

STOP SMOKING. I know it's easier said than done. Nicotine, the key part of tobacco, is thought to relax the esophageal sphincter, which means acid can move up in the wrong direction, leading to reflux and heartburn.

IF YOU GET REFLUX WHILE IN BED OR SLEEPING, try lying on your left side. Why? The esophagus is connected to the right side of the stomach, which means that lying on the left prevents the acid from being pushed back up the esophagus.

RAISE ONE END OF YOUR BED by 4 to 8 inches (10 to 20 cm) so that both your head and your chest are at a level just above your waist.

Other Strategies for Acid Reflux

NONSTEROIDAL ANTI-INFLAMMATORY DRUGS (NSAIDs) may make symptoms worse. The most common types include ibuprofen, aspirin, naproxen, and diclofenac. If you're unsure, check with your doctor or pharmacist.

TALK TO YOUR DOCTOR OR PHARMACIST ABOUT DIFFERENT TYPES OF OVER-THE-COUNTER MEDICATION. The most common include antacids, which help to neutralize the acid (available as a liquid or a chewable tablet, like Tums). Some antacids are also combined with alginates (e.g., Gaviscon); this forms a foam layer on top of your stomach contents, preventing the acid from moving back up the esophagus. There are also histamine H2-receptor antagonists (such as ranitidine) and proton-pump inhibitors (such as omeprazole), which decrease the production of stomach acid. If you're relying on over-the-counter medications at least twice a week for long periods, it's worth a visit to your doctor.

Exercise-Associated Gut Discomfort

Despite the many benefits of exercise, strenuous endurance activities can cause gut discomfort in many people. This can affect not only our enjoyment of exercise but also our ability to refuel while doing it, leading to impaired performance and delayed recovery. If you are currently struggling with exercise-associated gut discomfort, here are some strategies worth trying. Remember: Every gut is different, so do what works for you.

- **HYDRATION:** Ensure you are well hydrated before starting exercise (which means paying attention to your thirst both the day before and on the day) and continue to hydrate during exercise when possible. It's difficult to put a figure on how much you need to drink; instead, current recommendations suggest a "drink to thirst" approach is the best way to maintain optimal hydration around exercise. For exercise lasting under two hours, water will suffice but, for longer events, a standard sports drink that contains electrolytes might be better.

- **PRE-EVENT DIET:** If you've experienced exercise-associated gut discomfort before, try restricting the key higher-FODMAP foods (see table on page 159) from your diet between twenty-four and forty-eight hours prior to strenuous endurance training and/or events. There is growing evidence to suggest that restricting these foods (or a more formal low-FODMAP diet, as discussed on page 155) before an event may benefit those prone to exercise-associated gut discomfort, reducing symptoms both during and after exercise. That said, reintroducing these foods after the event is important to support good overall gut health. Visit a registered sports dietitian for individualized support.

- **PRE-EXERCISE MEAL:** Everyone's digestion is different, but having your last main meal between two and four hours before strenuous endurance training and/or an event is likely to decrease gut discomfort. If you do have a snack closer to the exercise, opt for foods lower in fiber, protein, and fat because these will be more rapidly digested (decreasing the potential for gut discomfort when starting the exercise). My go-to snack is an English muffin with jam and half a ripe banana.

- **DURING EXERCISE:** Training the gut to tolerate feeding during exercise is an important part of training for endurance events lasting longer than two hours. Why two hours? This is, on average, how long our body's energy stores can sustain exercise of at least a moderate intensity. It's best to incorporate nutrition training into your training program to increase gut tolerance and reduce the risk of symptoms. High-carbohydrate, low-fiber options are best for eating during exercise.

If you are struggling with underlying gut symptoms and are new to exercise, start with lower-impact exercise, such as power walking, cycling, cross-training machines, or swimming, and build up the duration and intensity over several months.

As we come to the end of what I consider the "bread and butter" of gut complaints, I hope you're feeling more informed and confident to tackle those bothersome symptoms as they arise. For those with one or two mild or moderate gut symptoms, you may find this chapter is enough to rid yourself of them entirely. For others with more complex issues or stubborn symptoms, you may need a little extra support and some more investigation, which we'll walk through step by step in the coming chapters. That said, it's worth keeping an open mind—I've had many patients with debilitating symptoms regain complete control of their lives with the strategies outlined in this chapter alone. This is why I encourage everyone to start here. Even if it's not successful, it's never a waste of time; think of it instead as taking you a step closer to finding the right strategies for you and your gut. Don't worry, we're here to work it out between you two.

CHAPTER 5

Food Intolerances

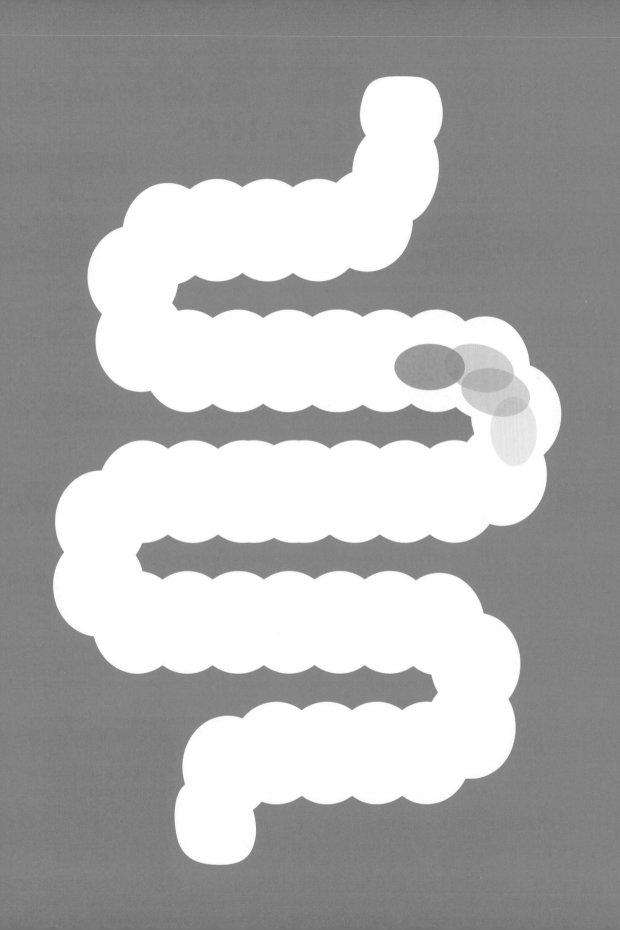

Food Intolerances

Most of my patients associate their gut symptoms with eating. But once we delve a little deeper, it's only a few who turn out to have food-specific symptoms such as food intolerance. So how do you know whether a specific food or component really doesn't agree with you or whether there's actually another cause for your gut symptoms, such as irritable bowel syndrome (IBS)? I'm not going to tell you it's straightforward, because it's not, but what makes it more difficult is all the unnecessary confusion on this topic. As a result, people tend to exclude various foods with no real coherent plan, and this can end up doing more harm than good.

One of my patients, thirty-one-year-old Stephanie, recently suffered the damaging consequences that can occur when this happens. Stephanie had been battling gut issues since her high school days, but after giving birth recently, her symptoms had become so bad that she was no longer able to control her bowels and, after an embarrassing incident, she was scared to leave the house. At her wits' end, Stephanie turned to online forums in a desperate attempt to resolve her debilitating symptoms. Following online advice, Stephanie began excluding different food groups such as whole grains and dairy. Week by week, she found herself cutting out more and more suspected food culprits, until she was down to just twelve "safe" foods. By this stage, she had become so dangerously thin that her milk supply had stopped, her once-lustrous hair had become thin and dull, her thoughts were foggy, and she was on the verge of being too weak to care for her baby. At rock bottom, she came to see me in my clinic. We sat together and went through her journey and, halfway through, it became abundantly clear to me that Stephanie's symptoms weren't the result of any food intolerance. Instead, she had a severe case of IBS that was being perpetuated by anxiety and malnutrition.

Yes, Stephanie's case was extreme but, sadly, this type of downward spiral with suspected food intolerances is something I see all too often.

This chapter will help cut through the confusion, equipping you with the tools and confidence to safely determine whether or not a specific food may be causing your gut symptoms.

There are two main types of food hypersensitivities: food intolerances and food aller-gies. Although this chapter will focus on food intolerances, it's worth knowing a little more about allergies, too, because the two conditions are often confused with each other. Unlike food intolerances, food allergies involve the immune system, where the body mistakenly tags specific food proteins as harmful. In turn, this triggers the body's defense system. As a result, the symptoms associated with a food allergy are typically more severe than those with food intolerances and can include difficulty breathing, a racing heart rate, and skin rashes, as well as digestive issues. Food allergies are less common, affecting around 1 to 2 percent of adults, and should be diagnosed only by a qualified clinician. The most common food allergens are cow's milk, egg, wheat, soy, nuts, seeds, and fish, although most allergies are outgrown in early childhood. In adults, the most common form of food allergy is oral allergy syndrome (see below). Another condition that may be considered a type of food hypersensitivity is celiac disease. Although it involves the immune system, it's not actually an allergy but is instead an autoimmune condition where, when exposed to gluten (a protein found in grains like wheat), the body's defense system attacks the intestine.

Food intolerances are far more common than food allergies and celiac disease combined, affecting as many as 20 percent of adults. Although they're not life-threatening, food intolerances can significantly affect your quality of life as well as your relationship with food, so it's worth getting on top of them.

Oral Allergy Syndrome (OAS)

Oral allergy syndrome (OAS), also known as pollen-food syndrome or pollen fruit syndrome (PFS), is the single most common type of food allergy in adults. Typically, the symptoms are immediate and include mild itching, tingling, or swelling of the tongue and lips. Those who get hay fever in the spring are more likely to have OAS because their body mistakes the culprit food proteins for pollen proteins and sets up an allergic response. Foods most likely to trigger symptoms include apple, kiwi, peaches, plums, carrots, Brazil nuts, walnuts, strawberries, hazelnuts, and almonds. Interestingly, cooking or processing foods (e.g., canning them) may improve tolerance. This is because heating the food breaks down the protein molecules and makes them inactive so they no longer trigger an allergic reaction. Symptoms may also be relieved with antihistamines. Thankfully, OAS is not life-threatening, and many people live happy, healthy lives with OAS without even realizing they have it. If you suspect you have it and it's bothering you, visit your healthcare professional, who can provide further guidance on diagnosis and management.

Is It a Food Intolerance?

With the growing awareness of gut disorders like IBS, it's increasingly common for people to jump to the conclusion that their gut problem must be IBS, without considering whether their symptoms are the result of a food intolerance (the opposite of Stephanie's case). In such instances, food intolerances are left undiagnosed, which leads to ineffective management and ongoing suffering. This is why it's worth ruling out common food intolerances as a cause of your gut symptoms first. The good news is it's something you can get started with at home, using my simple 3R Method.

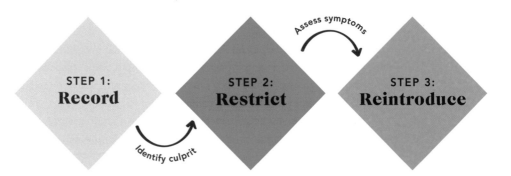

Before we start, I want you to remember all the good that food does for us: It gives us energy to follow our dreams and provides us with vital nutrients for our brain, hair, skin, and teeth. When talking about food intolerances, it can be easy to develop negative thoughts about food. The purpose of this chapter is to counter this; it's about developing your confidence and enabling you to regain the simple pleasure of eating by teaching you how to safely identify or discount a food intolerance, and so avoid unnecessary restrictions.

When it comes to symptoms, food intolerances can be expressed in other areas besides the gut; they may also affect the skin, airways, muscles, and joints and can cause headaches and fatigue. However, gut symptoms are by far the most common and will be our main focus in this chapter.

The Challenges

Identifying specific food intolerances is not always straightforward. To help you become a better food intolerance "detective," it will be useful for you to understand some of the main challenges, particularly when it comes to interpreting your results from Step 1: Record.

- **CHALLENGE 1:** Food is complex. Food components that can cause reactions are often naturally present in (or added to) a wide range of foods, and meals contain multiple ingredients. To help you overcome this challenge, I've developed tables detailing which foods and drinks contain commonly suspected culprits. If after Step 1: Record (see page 127) you're still not able to identify a food trigger using these tables but feel your symptoms are related to a food intolerance, it's possible that there's more than one culprit (although this is much less common). If this is the case, it's worth discussing your findings with a trained food detective: a dietitian.

- **CHALLENGE 2:** Unlike food allergies, food intolerances are often dose-dependent. This means most people with food intolerances can tolerate a portion of the food culprit. The amount (your tolerance threshold) also differs from person to person.

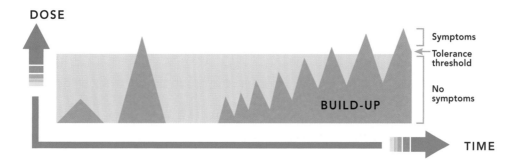

- **CHALLENGE 3:** Timing of symptoms. Symptoms experienced during or immediately after eating may have nothing to do with that meal. Instead, they may be related to an earlier meal. How? As we touched on in chapter 1, when food enters the stomach, it triggers movement in the large intestine, known as the gastrocolic reflex. This process helps to move previous meals through the large intestine, making them available to our hungry gut microbiota (GM). For some intolerances, this mechanism may trigger symptoms. But for some people with IBS, it might simply be the size of the meal that triggers gut symptoms and might have nothing to do with the actual food. What's more, the effect may be heightened, depending on your stress levels that day.

The Common Culprits

Below, we'll address the most commonly reported food intolerances that can lead to gut symptoms, including lactose (milk sugar), wheat, and gluten. We'll also touch on others that you may have come across, including fructose (fruit sugar), caffeine, histamine, and sulfite intolerances.

Lactose

Lactose is a unique carbohydrate found only in milk from mammals: cow, goat, sheep, buffalo, and human breast milk. Without wanting to bring back dreaded memories of high school chemistry: Lactose is made up of two sugars, glucose and galactose. For lactose to be absorbed from the intestine and into your bloodstream, it needs to be broken down into these two single sugars. This is the job of an enzyme called lactase, which is found on the lining of the small intestine. A large percentage of adults don't make enough lactase, and therefore the lactose isn't absorbed efficiently in the small intestine, resulting in lactose intolerance. The prevalence of lactose intolerance varies widely between populations. For instance, lactase deficiency occurs in as few as 5 percent of North Europeans and North Americans of European origin, yet up to 90 percent of Asian, African, and Caribbean adult populations are affected.[33] Despite the high rates of lactase deficiency, only a subset of people actually experience gut upset and are therefore considered lactose intolerant. Why is that? For some, their GM is thought to make up for the lack of lactase enzymes in their body by efficiently metabolizing the lactose for them.

There is some evidence suggesting that other components in standard cow's milk—specifically, certain types of protein known as A1 and A2 beta-casein—may be poorly tolerated by some people. Early evidence suggests that milk with only A2 beta-casein may be better tolerated in a subset of people than milk containing a mix of the two proteins.[34] If you live in Europe, the United States, Australia, or New Zealand, your standard cow's milk typically comes from Holstein-Friesian (black-and-white) cows and contains a mix of the two proteins. In contrast, cows in other areas such as Africa and India (*Bos indicus*) produce only A2 protein in their milk. We'll explore milk intolerance more in Step 3: Reintroduction.

> ## Common Symptoms Associated with Lactose Intolerance
>
> - **LOOSE POOPS AND DIARRHEA**
>   *(NOTE: This is not always the case; some may get constipation.)*
>
> - **BLOATING**
>
> - **WIND**
>
> - **TUMMY PAIN**

Two Main Forms of Lactose Intolerance

PRIMARY LACTASE DEFICIENCY: This is the inherited form and typically presents between the ages of five and twenty years as lactase production decreases. This is the more common form of lactose intolerance.

SECONDARY LACTASE DEFICIENCY: As a result of a gut illness or damage to the small intestine, there is a loss of lactase production, meaning there are fewer enzymes available to digest the lactose. This leads to malabsorption. Examples of causes include gut infections, undiagnosed celiac disease, and active Crohn's disease. The good news is that most often this type is short term. Within a few months, once the intestine has healed, the levels of lactase in the body return to normal.

Wheat and Gluten

Wheat is often the first thing to be excluded when people suspect a food intolerance. Although it's certainly not as common as suggested online, there are several wheat-related culprits that people may react to, and guess what? It's not only gluten. It's true that some people struggle to digest gluten, but there are other types of components in wheat, including wheat germ agglutinin, amylase trypsin inhibitors, and fructans, that may trigger people's symptoms. In fact, researchers have suggested that non-celiac gluten sensitivity (NCGS) may be more accurately termed non-celiac wheat sensitivity (NCWS), because it's not always the gluten component of wheat that people are struggling with. The jury is still out.

Why am I telling you this? I don't have a soft spot for gluten and I certainly don't want to complicate the matter, but it's worth knowing that, if you react to wheat, it may not be gluten but other components that are causing you grief. This means that not only could you be unnecessarily restricting your diet by using a gluten-free approach, but also that you won't completely shake your symptoms if the true culprit remains in your diet. This concept was demonstrated in a study where people with self-diagnosed NCGS already on a gluten-free diet further benefited when fructans (which are also found in gluten-free foods) were restricted.[35] This is something I often see in my clinic, too.

One case that particularly springs to mind is that of twenty-two-year-old James. James had self-diagnosed NCGS and, as a result, was following a strict gluten-free diet. As soon as he walked into my clinic room I could see by his hunched shoulders and negative expression that he was feeling defeated. He sat down and shared at length the hurdles he'd had to overcome to go gluten-free, including the social isolation—for example, he was no longer able to drink beer with his friends, since standard beer contains gluten. Despite all this effort, his gut symptoms persisted. Together, we went through his diet, and I noticed he was consuming very large amounts of fructans, specifically from onion and garlic (fructans are a type of fermentable carbohydrate found in wheat, onions, garlic, and many fruits and vegetables; we'll cover this in chapter 6). James's symptoms suggested that he was suffering from classic IBS, so I asked him if he would be willing to cut out the onion and garlic for two weeks and report back. I could see he was a little hesitant to further restrict his diet, but after I explained the potential mechanisms (he was studying science, after all), he was on board. Two weeks later, I received an email from a very happy James—it had worked: His bowels, which he'd been suffering with for over three years, were no longer unruly. I did make sure that James came back to discuss reintroducing gluten-containing foods, as well as onion and garlic and other high-fructan foods, once he had better control of his IBS—oh, and the beer was back on the "menu": We did have a chat about responsible drinking, too, of course!

TAKE-HOME MESSAGE: *Don't assume it's gluten and cut all sources from your diet before considering alternative causes. Step 1 in the 3R Method (see page 127) can help you objectively assess this.*

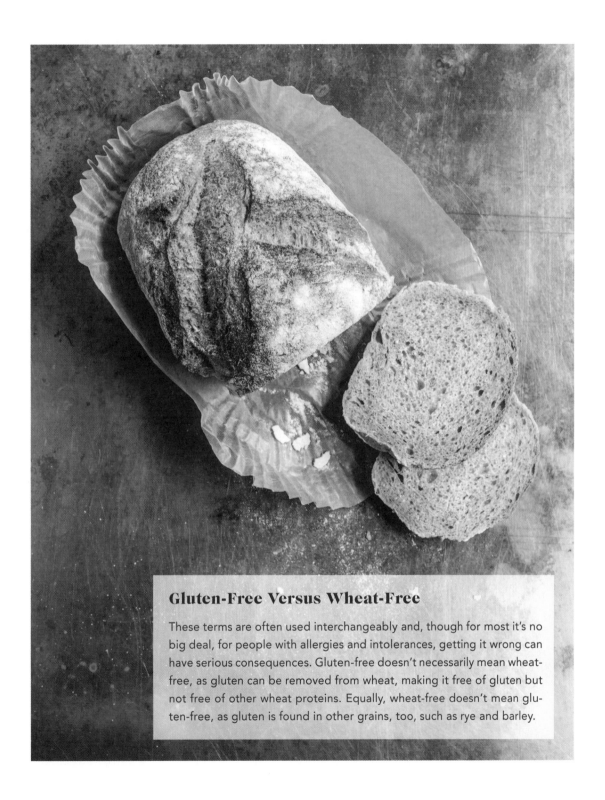

Gluten-Free Versus Wheat-Free

These terms are often used interchangeably and, though for most it's no big deal, for people with allergies and intolerances, getting it wrong can have serious consequences. Gluten-free doesn't necessarily mean wheat-free, as gluten can be removed from wheat, making it free of gluten but not free of other wheat proteins. Equally, wheat-free doesn't mean gluten-free, as gluten is found in other grains, too, such as rye and barley.

Fructose

Fructose is one of the sugars naturally found in fruit and honey. It's also increasingly being added to sweeten other food and drinks in the form of high-fructose corn syrup, particularly in the US. Unlike the milk sugar lactose, the fruit sugar fructose is a single unit, so it doesn't need to be digested by enzymes before being absorbed into the body. On face value, you may think this means absorption is unlimited, but there's a catch: There's a quota limiting the amount of fructose that gets in at each sitting—think of it as similar to admissions into a theater. Beyond this quota, the excess fructose has no choice but to travel onward into the large intestine, bringing with it a load of extra fluid, and is rapidly fermented by our GM. Interestingly, most of us cannot absorb large amounts of fructose in a single sitting. This explains why, when you can't stop eating those juicy cherries, even those of us with strong guts may experience some bloating and loose poops. For a subset of people, smaller amounts of fructose can trigger these gut symptoms. Nonetheless, fructose intolerance on its own is thought to be rather rare. Instead, for those with IBS, fructose forms part of a collection of fermentable carbohydrates known as FODMAPs, which, in moderate amounts, may trigger symptoms in some (we'll discuss these on page 153). The good news is, if glucose is also present in the food, as in the case of most fruits, it will help your body absorb the fructose (opening a second viewing room, in the theater metaphor). This is why, although all fruits contain fructose, some are better tolerated than others in people who are more sensitive, as we'll discuss when we address FODMAPs. It's also worth noting that, once you get your IBS under control, you can likely enjoy higher-fructose foods without any issues.

Histamine Intolerance

This can cause a range of symptoms beyond the gut. Histamine intolerance may mimic an allergic reaction, so allergies should be ruled out first. It can be difficult to diagnose histamine intolerance, as diet isn't the only source; our body and GM can also produce histamine. Foods high in histamines include aged and fermented food and drinks (e.g., cheese, sauerkraut, alcoholic drinks, and cured meats); most fish, including smoked and canned; fruit, such as oranges and bananas; some vegetables, such as spinach; and legumes such as fava beans.

Sulfite Sensitivity

Sulfite is primarily used as a preservative in a range of foods, including dried fruit, processed meats, and drinks. They're also naturally present in fermented grape products (i.e., wine and vinegar). People with asthma seem to have a higher risk of sensitivity. Symptoms are not gut specific and can include hives, flushing, wheezing, and a stuffy nose.

Caffeine

Although most adults can consume up to 400 milligrams of caffeine a day without side effects (200 mg in pregnancy), some people are more sensitive due to genetics and how their bodies break it down. The most common side effects include nervousness, anxiety, insomnia, and gut symptoms. Although we typically associate caffeine with coffee, there are many other sources of caffeine outlined in the table below. The caffeine content isn't typically declared on food and drink labels, making it difficult to know exactly how much you are consuming. What makes it even more tricky is that with naturally occurring sources, such as coffee and tea, the caffeine content can vary according to the plant variety, growing conditions, and brewing method. Keep this in mind when you're playing food detective.

Caffeine Content of Common Products

BEVERAGE (serving size)	RANGE (mg)	AVERAGE (mg)
Tea		
Black (8 ounces/240 ml)	25–110	50
Green (8 ounces/240 ml)	30–50	45
Brewed (8 ounces/240 ml)	40–120	55
Coffee		
Decaffeinated (8 ounces/240 ml)	5–10	5
Instant (8 ounces/240 ml)	25–175	95
Brewed (8 ounces/240 ml)	100–200	135
Espresso (2 ounces/60 ml)	60–180	80
Dark chocolate 70 percent (50 g)	–	40
Cola (11 ounces/330 ml)	10–70	40
Energy drink (17 ounces/500 ml)	55–175	160
Cold or flu medication	15–200	see package

Source: Nutrition Bulletin[36]

Risky Business

Before we get into the 3R Method, it would be remiss of me not to highlight the risks associated with a restricted diet. Not only can long-term food restriction be socially isolating, but cutting out food groups can also displace other nutrients in your diet. Take, for instance, restricting gluten. An observational study of close to 200,000 people (without celiac disease) demonstrated that those with the highest gluten consumption (the top 20 percent) had a 20 percent lower risk of developing type 2 diabetes, compared to those with the lowest gluten intake (the bottom 20 percent).[37] The researchers were able to explain this finding, at least in part, by the fact that those who cut gluten also tended to eat less grain fiber, which is known to protect against type 2 diabetes. What about our GM? It's affected, too. For instance, a gluten-free diet has been shown to decrease bacteria known to produce those beneficial short-chain fatty acids.

Still not convinced? Researchers have shown that not only were gluten-free foods 159 percent more expensive, but they also, on average, contained more added sugar and salt, and less fiber and protein than their gluten-containing alternatives. Now, of course, opting for more whole foods and fewer processed options (e.g., choosing gluten-free oats instead of ultra-processed gluten-free cereals) can help to avoid this when going gluten-free. It does, however, highlight the need to be more aware of the ways in which other aspects of your diet can be affected if you cut foods out. Long-term food restriction may also lead to greater sensitivity to certain foods. Considering all these factors, it becomes rather apparent that restricting your diet when you don't need to may do more harm than good.

 Caution: *If you have a history of disordered eating, please seek support from a dietitian before considering the 3R Method.*

Diagnosing Intolerances

The gold standard for diagnosing food intolerances is an elimination diet, followed by a placebo-controlled reintroduction. These describe Step 2 and Step 3 in the 3R Method, respectively. This is based on a simple rationale: Restriction of the food in question should resolve your symptoms, and reintroduction should reproduce symptoms.

When it comes to Step 3, it's recommended that this is done blind, which means that you are unaware if you are eating the challenge food or a placebo (a food without the suspected culprit). This comes back to the gut-brain axis. Remember: The communication between the two is bidirectional, meaning the gut can influence the brain, and vice versa. Studies have shown that if we perceive that we have a food intolerance, our brain can send messages to our gut, inducing gut symptoms when we eat the suspected culprit. This phenomenon is known as the nocebo effect—the ability of negative expectations to manifest physical symptoms. Need the science to convince you? Don't worry: I did, too. A systematic review (in which scientists pool together the results from all the trials on one topic) found that 40 percent of people with a self-reported intolerance to gluten had similar or increased symptoms during the placebo (i.e., gluten-free) intervention, because they believed it contained gluten. It's similar to when we are mentally stressed or nervous: It can physically manifest in gut symptoms, despite our diet not changing. These findings reinforce why we shouldn't underestimate the power of our thoughts.

Invalid Food Tolerances

Despite the convincing marketing claims, there is no valid test for food intolerances (with lactose being the exception). Some of the common invalid tests to watch out for include IgG tests, hair analysis, and muscle analysis (kinesiology). Many of these tests attach themselves to scientific concepts that sound rather convincing. Take, for instance, the IgG test. This test involves exposing a sample of your blood to different foods and measuring the resulting antibody (IgG). The test claims this is a marker of "intolerance." Sounds pretty legit, right? The thing is, unlike IgE, which are valid for diagnosing certain allergies, most of us will actually develop IgG antibodies to food during our lifetime, despite not getting symptoms. This, explains expert immunologist Dr. Jenna Macciochi, is because IgG is an indicator of repeated exposure, not food intolerance.[38]

The 3R Method

There's no denying that food intolerances can be confusing to navigate, which is why the medical guidelines recommend seeing a dietitian. But having worked in healthcare for many years, I know access to a dietitian isn't always straightforward, with long waiting lists and high costs, which can be a deterrent for many. For those with only mild symptoms, it may also seem like a little too much as a first step. So what do we instinctively do? Turn to Google, of course. The outcome? Conflicting advice, long-term over-restriction, and persisting symptoms as you're sucked into a downhill spiral, like Stephanie. The answer? I'm going to be straight and tell you there's no quick fix. But there's a more effective and safer way of going about it: the 3R Method. This is something I developed with you in mind. The purpose is to provide you with the evidence-based tools needed to start the detective work safely at home. It's also the framework I regularly use in my clinic, as was the case with thirty-one-year-old Karen.

Karen had been suffering with bloating, loose poops, and bowel urgency since her early twenties. She explained that she'd recently been told that she had IBS and, after reading about the benefits of a low-FODMAP diet, she wanted to give it a try. I did my normal workup and found that Karen didn't fulfill the criteria for IBS (we'll discuss this more in chapter 6). Furthermore, from her brief diet history (her two-year-old son was getting a little impatient with us), I discovered that Karen's diet was really rather low in FODMAPs. I explained these findings to her, along with the complexity of the low-FODMAP diet, and suggested instead that, as a first step, we investigate whether a food tolerance could be the cause. Karen was, not surprisingly, a little relieved at not having to follow a strict diet. She also explained that she'd considered dairy and gluten intolerance over the years, but cutting them out never seemed to solve things. I asked Karen to complete Step 1: Record and return in a few weeks.

STEP 1:
Record

In order for you to play food detective, you'll need to collect some objective information. This involves recording a detailed diary for seven days, or two weeks if symptoms are less frequent, as outlined on page 129. If you're confident that you've already identified a food culprit, then you can move straight to Step 2.

During Step 1, try to keep your diet and lifestyle as normal as you can. The purpose is to identify whether anything you normally eat or do is causing the problem. If you can, record things in real time for the most accurate results. This way, you remember to include all the details (for example, that bite of your friend's burger you took or the leftover chips you snagged from your staff meeting). To help with this, it's a good idea to carry a notebook with you (or use a smartphone tracker app).

Main Sources of Commonly Reported Food Intolerances

• LACTOSE: Milk from animals, soft cheeses, yogurt, and milk-based desserts, e.g., custard and ice cream.

• WHEAT: All types (e.g., durum, farro, spelt, einkorn, Kamut, and triticale) and forms (e.g., semolina, couscous) of wheat.

• GLUTEN: All foods containing rye, wheat, or barley (e.g., breakfast cereals, bread, pizza, pasta, cake), and beer, barley water, and malted drinks.

My Gut Diary

This diary is designed to capture your gut symptoms, along with the key factors that can influence them, such as diet, mood, sleep, pooping habits, and other activities. The more accurate your diary is, the more helpful it will be in getting on top of your gut symptoms. You might like to use the diary template on page 130 (you'll also find this template at theguthealthdoctor.com/book) or just use a small notebook. Some tips for completing it appear on page 129.

Karen returned three weeks later, having dutifully completed her gut diary—it was time to play food detective. Her symptoms were worse during the week, on days she had a wheat-based breakfast cereal (with soy milk). From her diary, I could also see that each time she'd eaten a chocolate bar or custard, she'd have bowel urgency within an hour. After piecing together the information, I suspected that it was lactose. But what about her breakfast—she was using lactose-free milk after all? Unknown to Karen, her breakfast cereal wasn't lactose-free, as it contained powdered milk (a marketing trick to boost the protein and sweetness). I also noticed that she was taking a high-dose vitamin C supplement (she'd read it was a flu preventative).

With these clues noted, Karen moved on to Step 2, implementing three changes: 1) cutting out high-lactose foods (see page 135); 2) stopping her vitamin C supplement (which can cause gut upset in high doses); and 3) increasing her fruit intake (high in vitamin C) to two pieces spread across the day (Karen had cut out fruit, as she'd heard it was high in sugar and caused candida overgrowth—I happily busted that myth for her).

Example of How to Complete ◆

Day: Friday

Date: January 1, 2021

1. **DIET:** Write down everything you eat and drink along with the time (remember to record easily forgotten things like chewing gum, supplements, medication, total fluid intake, and so on). Try to be specific, including condiments like sauces and spreads, how the food was cooked (e.g., fried or raw), and estimated portions (no need to get the scales out).

2. **EXERCISE:** Record all forms of exercise, including power walking, gut-directed yoga, meditation, etc.

3. **POOPING HABITS:** As in Checking In with Your Poop (see page 24), record as much information as you can, including the time, consistency (type 1 to 7), color, approximate size, and any other notable characteristics, such as pieces of food or mucus.

4. **STRESSORS AND EMOTIONS:** Record any stressors, such as work meetings or family arguments, as well as your general mood throughout the day.

5. **GUT SYMPTOMS:** Record details of any gut symptoms, including the time they started, the time they ended, and the severity. Use the scale 1 (mild) to 5 (severe) to capture the severity.

6. **SLEEP:** Note your waking time and bedtime, and rate how refreshed you feel on a scale of 1 (super refreshed) to 5 (very groggy).

	MORNING
DIET	**6:45 am** 1/2 cup (50 g) rolled oats cooked with 3/4 cup plus 1 tablespoon (200 ml) soy milk. 1/2 banana and 1 tablespoon mixed seeds. 10 ounces (300 ml) water with probiotic **11:30 am** 1/2 slice of sourdough (whole wheat) with 1 tablespoon peanut butter
EXERCISE (physical and mental)	**6:20 am** Gut-directed yoga flow (10 minutes)
POOPING HABITS	**7:30 am** Type 3, brown, medium
STRESSORS AND EMOTIONS	**9:30 am** Stuck in traffic; frustrated **10:05 am** Late to meeting; embarrassed
GUT SYMPTOMS	Began 9:45 am Tummy pain (1) Bloating (3) Went for a walk and let out some wind—symptom improved by 11:20 a.m.
SLEEP	Wake: 6:00 am (2) Bedtime: 10:00 pm

Day: Date:	MORNING	AFTERNOON	EVENING
DIET			
EXERCISE (physical and mental)			
POOPING HABITS			
STRESSORS AND EMOTIONS			
GUT SYMPTOMS			
SLEEP			

Now it's your turn to play detective using your diary.
Follow the flow diagram below to determine the next step for you.

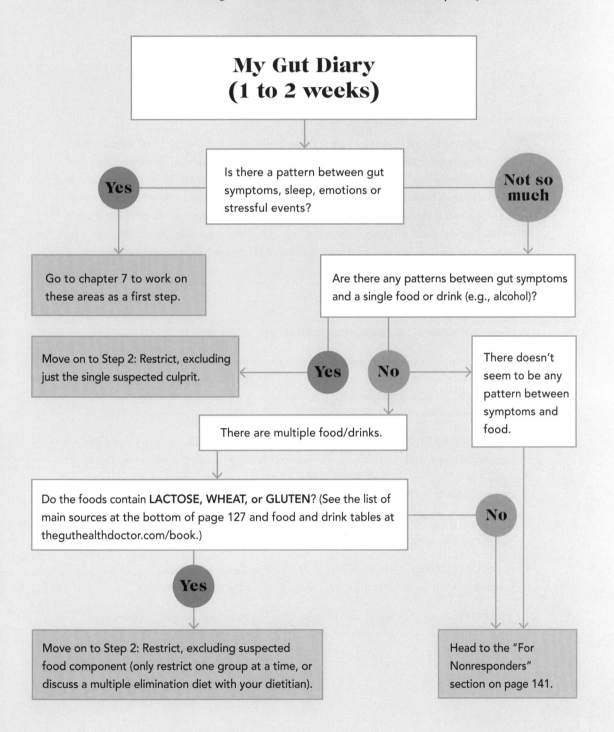

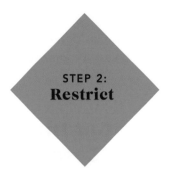

STEP 2:
Restrict

So your suspected food culprit (or culprits) has been identified—what next? As discussed earlier, the more you restrict your diet, the greater the nutritional risk. Therefore, if you've identified multiple food culprits (e.g., lactose and wheat), I recommend that you see a dietitian who can help guide you through restricting several food components at once. Also, remember: If you suspect an issue with gluten or wheat, it's best to see your doctor to be tested for celiac disease before excluding it from your diet. Why? You need to include a considerable amount of gluten in the diet for at least six weeks in order for your celiac test to be valid.

Preparation Is Key

Restricting common foods can take some planning.

- TIME: Choose a convenient period. Avoiding busy times at work and peak social seasons will make it easier to stick to the restrictions. If you do eat the food by mistake or for social reasons, it's completely OK. Just know that you may have residual symptoms for up to three days or so.

- KNOWLEDGE: Take a week or so to become familiar with dietary sources and the suggested alternative foods to ensure your diet is still nutritionally adequate. This is not a "detox" or weight-loss diet; you should still be meeting all your nutritional requirements and not excluding whole food groups.

- CLEAN OUT AND RESTOCK: Donate to a food bank or use up any foods you plan to restrict, and buy the replacements instead.

- HABIT FORMING: Get into the habit of checking labels before you buy, and consider planning meals for your first week to help ease yourself into it.

- SUPPORT: Keep your family and friends in the loop so they can help support you.

Before you remove the suspected culprit from your diet, use the Gut Feelings assessment on page 21 to assess your symptoms. Now, it's time to begin the restriction. If your symptoms resolve after two weeks, you can move straight on to Step 3—there's no need to wait. If, by week four, your symptoms have improved slightly, you may wish to continue up to of six weeks before moving on to Step 3. If your symptoms don't improve at all after four weeks, or only slightly after six weeks, it is best to put the eliminated food back into your diet and return to your usual diet. From there, head to page 141—Step 3 is not relevant to your situation.

So how did Karen get on? Her symptoms vanished after just one week. She couldn't believe it was that "simple." She was kicking herself for not having taken a more systematic approach when dealing with her initial suspicion of a food intolerance. The next step was reintroducing and, although she was a little apprehensive, Karen understood it was best to confirm it really was the lactose and high-dose vitamin C causing the problem. Karen challenged them one by one.

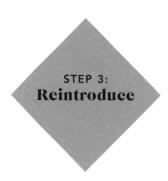

STEP 3:
Reintroduce

This step is essential to confirm whether the suspect food component really is the cause of your gut symptoms and not just an innocent bystander. It will also help you determine your tolerance threshold. If you have any concerns that it is an allergy, see your doctor or allergy specialist first and do not reintroduce. For those tempted to skip this section and just restrict the food long-term, here are some points worth considering.

- UNNECESSARILY OVER-RESTRICTING YOUR DIET INCREASES YOUR RISK OF MALNUTRITION, which occurs when your body doesn't get enough nutrients to maintain itself and your muscles start to waste away. This can leave you feeling tired and more likely to catch the flu, among many other things.

- COMPLETE RESTRICTION OVER A LONG PERIOD OF TIME MAY INCREASE YOUR SENSITIVITY AND LOWER YOUR TOLERANCE THRESHOLD. AS A CONSEQUENCE, symptoms may increase in severity when you accidentally eat those foods. I often see this with lactose intolerance.

- A LONG-TERM RESTRICTED DIET IS LINKED WITH A REDUCED FOOD-RELATED QUALITY OF LIFE. It reduces the fun of eating and socializing—and nobody wants that.

- MANY OF THESE FOODS ARE YOUR GM'S FAVORITES, which means that you could be denying not only your taste buds but your GM, too.

> **Caution:** *If you've been avoiding a food group for several years and have history of atopic symptoms (i.e., eczema, asthma, or hay fever), it is recommended that reintroduction is conducted by an allergy-specialist dietitian or an allergist.*

As we touched on earlier, the reintroduction process is most accurate when you are blind to the food—you don't know whether you're having the "active/challenge" food or the placebo test food. How to go about doing this, including test foods and amounts, is described in the flow diagrams on the next few pages. If you have identified a single food or drink culprit, follow the diagram on pages 138 to 139, using this as your "test food." On day one, start with one third of your normal portion, and increase by one third each day as appropriate. For the blind test, you'll need to get your family or a friend on board. Ask them to disguise the food so you can't tell the difference between the active and the placebo. Blending, toasting, or breading can be helpful ways to blind you—but be sure they don't add in any other suspected culprits! Before you are unblinded, complete both active and placebo challenges, even if you get symptoms with the first challenge. If you do get symptoms, wait until you are symptom-free again (usually up to three days) before moving on to the other test food. I get that it's not always possible to do food challenges blinded, so don't let that stop you from completing Step 3.

Lactose Content of Milk and Dairy Products

TYPE	PERCENT BY WEIGHT
Cow's milk	4.5
Condensed milk	12.5
Powdered milk	53.0
Goat's milk	4.5
Sheep's milk	5.0
Cream	2.0
Crème fraîche	2.5
Firm cheese (e.g., cheddar)	2.5–7.0
Processed cheese (e.g., cheese spread)	Less than 1.0
Cottage cheese	4.5–7.5
Yogurt	3.0
Ice cream	4.5
Rice pudding	5.0
Custard	4.0
Chocolate (milk, white)	5.0
Chocolate (dark, 70%)	9.0–10.0
Butter	Less than 1.0

Source: Nutrition Bulletin[39]

Testing Response to Lactose

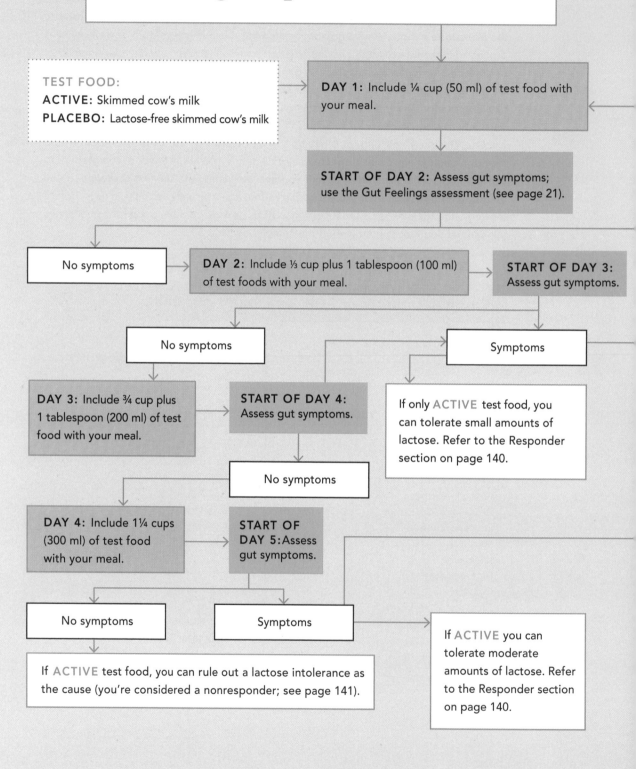

TEST FOOD:
ACTIVE: Skimmed cow's milk
PLACEBO: Lactose-free skimmed cow's milk

DAY 1: Include ¼ cup (50 ml) of test food with your meal.

START OF DAY 2: Assess gut symptoms; use the Gut Feelings assessment (see page 21).

No symptoms

DAY 2: Include ⅓ cup plus 1 tablespoon (100 ml) of test foods with your meal.

START OF DAY 3: Assess gut symptoms.

No symptoms

Symptoms

DAY 3: Include ¾ cup plus 1 tablespoon (200 ml) of test food with your meal.

START OF DAY 4: Assess gut symptoms.

If only **ACTIVE** test food, you can tolerate small amounts of lactose. Refer to the Responder section on page 140.

No symptoms

DAY 4: Include 1¼ cups (300 ml) of test food with your meal.

START OF DAY 5: Assess gut symptoms.

No symptoms

Symptoms

If **ACTIVE** test food, you can rule out a lactose intolerance as the cause (you're considered a nonresponder; see page 141).

If **ACTIVE** you can tolerate moderate amounts of lactose. Refer to the Responder section on page 140.

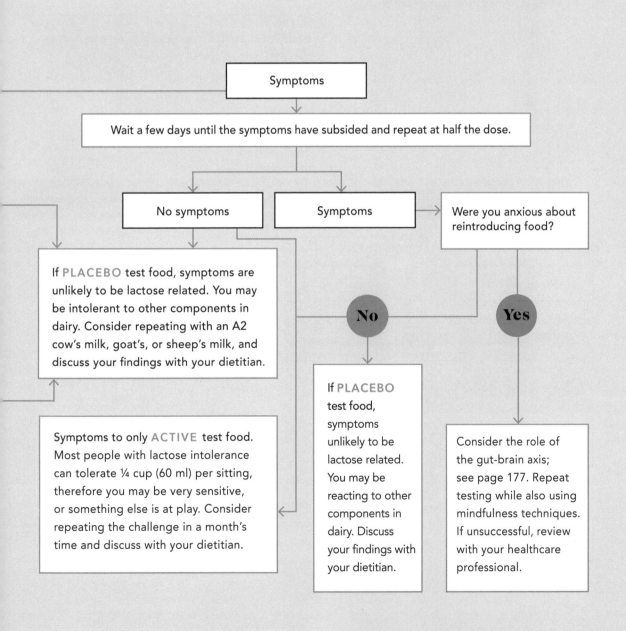

Continue a low lactose diet throughout the test period.

Symptoms

Wait a few days until the symptoms have subsided and repeat at half the dose.

No symptoms

Symptoms

Were you anxious about reintroducing food?

If PLACEBO test food, symptoms are unlikely to be lactose related. You may be intolerant to other components in dairy. Consider repeating with an A2 cow's milk, goat's, or sheep's milk, and discuss your findings with your dietitian.

No

Yes

Symptoms to only ACTIVE test food. Most people with lactose intolerance can tolerate ¼ cup (60 ml) per sitting, therefore you may be very sensitive, or something else is at play. Consider repeating the challenge in a month's time and discuss with your dietitian.

If PLACEBO test food, symptoms unlikely to be lactose related. You may be reacting to other components in dairy. Discuss your findings with your dietitian.

Consider the role of the gut-brain axis; see page 177. Repeat testing while also using mindfulness techniques. If unsuccessful, review with your healthcare professional.

Testing Response to Gluten/Wheat

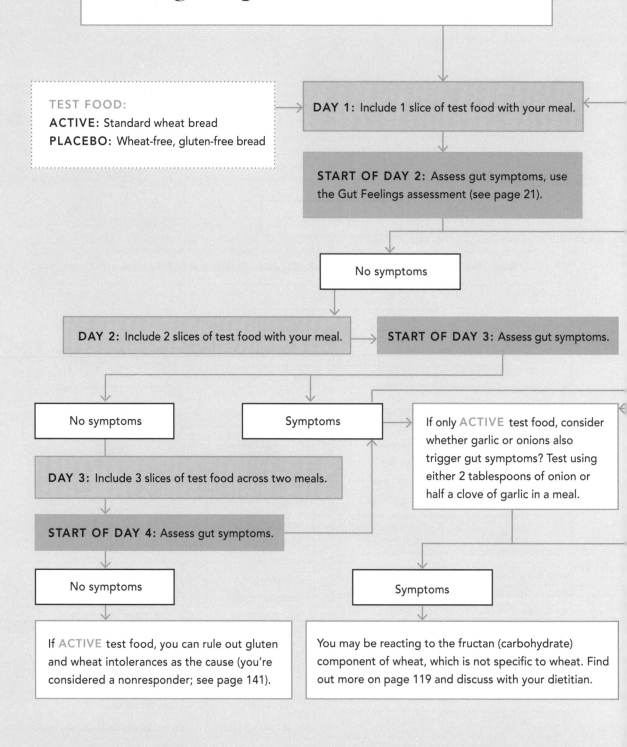

TEST FOOD:
ACTIVE: Standard wheat bread
PLACEBO: Wheat-free, gluten-free bread

DAY 1: Include 1 slice of test food with your meal.

START OF DAY 2: Assess gut symptoms, use the Gut Feelings assessment (see page 21).

No symptoms

DAY 2: Include 2 slices of test food with your meal.

START OF DAY 3: Assess gut symptoms.

No symptoms

Symptoms

If only **ACTIVE** test food, consider whether garlic or onions also trigger gut symptoms? Test using either 2 tablespoons of onion or half a clove of garlic in a meal.

DAY 3: Include 3 slices of test food across two meals.

START OF DAY 4: Assess gut symptoms.

No symptoms

Symptoms

If **ACTIVE** test food, you can rule out gluten and wheat intolerances as the cause (you're considered a nonresponder; see page 141).

You may be reacting to the fructan (carbohydrate) component of wheat, which is not specific to wheat. Find out more on page 119 and discuss with your dietitian.

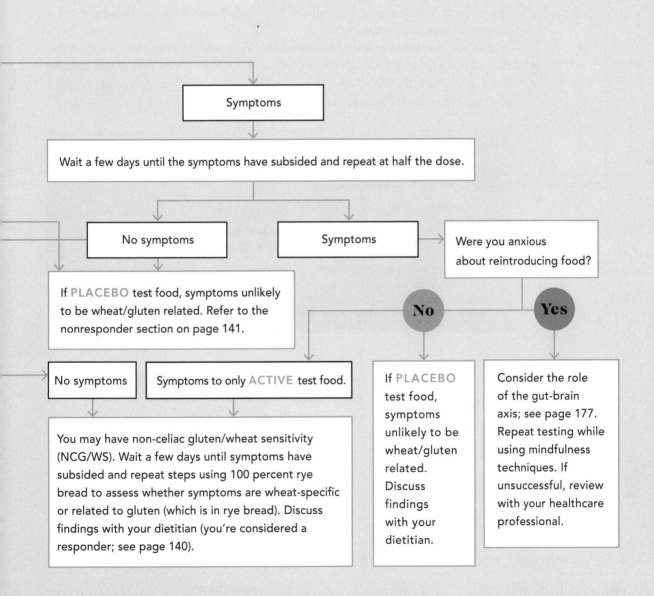

Continue a gluten-/wheat-free diet throughout the test period.

Symptoms

Wait a few days until the symptoms have subsided and repeat at half the dose.

No symptoms

Symptoms

Were you anxious about reintroducing food?

If PLACEBO test food, symptoms unlikely to be wheat/gluten related. Refer to the nonresponder section on page 141.

No

Yes

No symptoms

Symptoms to only ACTIVE test food.

If PLACEBO test food, symptoms unlikely to be wheat/gluten related. Discuss findings with your dietitian.

Consider the role of the gut-brain axis; see page 177. Repeat testing while using mindfulness techniques. If unsuccessful, review with your healthcare professional.

You may have non-celiac gluten/wheat sensitivity (NCG/WS). Wait a few days until symptoms have subsided and repeat steps using 100 percent rye bread to assess whether symptoms are wheat-specific or related to gluten (which is in rye bread). Discuss findings with your dietitian (you're considered a responder; see page 140).

What Next?

For the Responders

If it turns out that you're intolerant to one of the common culprits, keep in mind that it may not be forever. This is why reassessing your tolerances over time is a good idea. If you find that you can tolerate small amounts of the food, continue to include the foods up to your tolerance threshold (particularly for lactose). If you do feel it's necessary to exclude them completely, remember to nourish your body with the other sources of the key nutrients to ensure your diet remains balanced. If ever in doubt, be sure to see a dietitian or registered nutritionist.

Can you increase your tolerance threshold? There is some evidence to suggest you can, particularly for lactose, as outlined below. If you have issues with wheat, but also find that you have IBS (see chapter 6), you may find you can reintroduce larger portions of wheat once your IBS is under control.

Improving Tolerance to Lactose

- *Most can continue to eat small amounts throughout the day without symptoms (up to 12 grams of lactose per day).*

- *Consume as part of a meal rather than on its own.*

- *Consuming small amounts regularly may help increase your tolerance (possibly through adaptation of your GM—it may even act as a prebiotic).*

- *Fermented milk products, including plain probiotic yogurt and kefir, typically contain less lactose compared to equivalent unfermented forms, thanks to the microbes that eat some of it. Keep in mind that the amount varies, depending on the types of microbes and the time left to ferment.*

For Nonresponders

For those who didn't identify any food triggers, I know you may feel somewhat disheartened that you haven't gotten to the bottom of your issue at this stage, but please don't be. There are a number of positive outcomes that have resulted from going through this systematic process. First, if you were restricting foods, you should now be able to confidently reintroduce them, knowing that they aren't the cause. Second, for some, Step 1 may have helped you identify other non-diet-related triggers, such as stress, which can be managed by adopting the strategies we'll discuss in chapter 7. Third, ruling out these common food intolerances will put you in a better position to move on to chapter 6 and assess whether, as in Stephanie's case, IBS could be behind your symptoms. Fourth, if you still suspect a food intolerance, having gone through the three steps will make the next step (seeing your healthcare professional) much more efficient in helping you to identify what lies at the root of your gut issues. How? You've already completed the first-line strategies that your doctor or dietitian would normally spend the first appointment addressing, allowing them to move on to investigating more complex causes. Along with taking a completed My Gut Diary (see page 128) to your appointment, it's always a good idea to prepare yourself for the questions you may be asked in your appointment so you can get the most out of your time with them (see below).

- Do your symptoms follow a pattern (for example, are they always in the evening)?

- Have you had any previous tests or examinations?

- Are your symptoms affected by stress?

- How quickly after eating do you see a reaction?

- Do you have a family history of gut issues, allergies, or any other conditions?

- What is your most troublesome symptom?

- When did your symptoms first start?

- How often do you experience symptoms in a week or month?

- Are you on any medication or supplements? (Best to bring a list with you, if you are.)

- Do you suffer from any allergies (e.g., eczema, asthma, hay fever, animal hair, dust mites, other diagnosed food allergies)?

CHAPTER 6
Irritable Bowel Syndrome

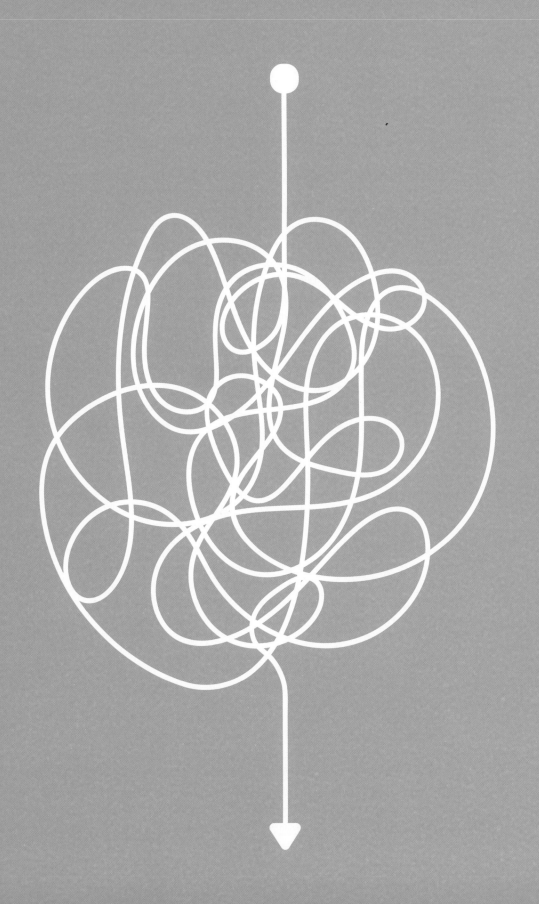

IBS

Do you suffer from several gut symptoms, including tummy pain? Having a collection of symptoms is extremely common, particularly in people with irritable bowel syndrome (IBS), a gut disorder that affects as many as one in ten adults worldwide.[40]

For many, IBS can be extremely debilitating. It can affect your work life with more time taken off sick, your social life with more canceled events, and your self-confidence, too, as it can cause bloating that rivals the size of a pregnant belly. What further adds to many people's frustration is the unpredictability and inability to control symptoms. Indeed, one study of nearly 2,000 IBS sufferers found that they would be willing to give up 25 percent of their remaining life span to be symptom-free[41]—reinforcing just how crippling the condition can be.

> I witnessed this level of despair in forty-one-year-old Jack. Over a two-year period, Jack had seen over fifteen different specialists, traveling across the country in a desperate attempt to cure his debilitating gut symptoms. He quit his job, re-mortgaged his house, and admitted that his pervasive suicidal thoughts may have ended with him taking his own life if it hadn't been for his supportive partner, who happened to be a psychologist.

While the severity of the symptoms varies from person to person, suffering from uncontrolled IBS should be a thing of the past. There are now international guidelines informing the management of IBS, along with breakthrough research, including work from my research team, that highlights the powerful role that diet can play.

For those with IBS, this chapter is about equipping you with the necessary information and tools to get you on the road to recovery, just as Jack was able to take control of his IBS. We will cover the evidence behind the syndrome, including what to expect, how to self-manage, and when you may need to call in the gut experts.

First Up, Is It IBS?

This seemingly simple question is actually quite tricky, because there's currently no specific test to diagnose IBS. Instead, it's a diagnosis you and your doctor come to after ruling out other diseases, such as celiac disease and inflammatory bowel disease (IBD), where symptoms often overlap with IBS (see the red flags on page 89). Thankfully, there are simple tests your doctor can perform to rule these out, which is why I always recommend paying them a visit before attributing your symptoms to IBS.

The Cause

IBS is considered a disorder of the gut-brain axis. This essentially means that the communication between the gut and the brain is out of whack. This is expressed through an overly sensitive intestine, which is more formally referred to as visceral hypersensitivity. As a result, there's an exaggerated response to various things, including fluctuating hormones, food and drinks, and medication. This explains why most people find their symptoms get worse with poor sleep, with stress, and after eating and drinking.

There is no single cause for IBS; several factors can increase your risk of getting it. One of the most well known is suffering from a gut infection like traveler's diarrhea or food poisoning: Your risk of getting IBS is over four times greater if you've had a gut infection in the previous year. It's also been suggested that, in addition to having a gut infection, your risk is further increased by your biological sex (it's higher in females), the severity of the infection, and a history of anxiety or depression. Interestingly, a history of trauma and chronic stress are additional risk factors for IBS. There may also be a genetic component to IBS, suggesting that some people are more susceptible than others, based on suspect genes linked to gut movement, gut "leakiness," and how sensitive your intestine is. It might be worth talking to your parents about whether they've ever suffered from IBS. That said, having specific genes doesn't mean you are destined for IBS; instead, it's determined by a combination of genes and your environment. For instance, stress (your environment) can affect whether IBS-related genes are "switched on."

Assessment: IS IT IBS OR ANOTHER FUNCTIONAL GUT DISORDER?

Complete the IBS assessment below to determine whether you might have IBS or another functional gut disorder.

Once the overlapping conditions are ruled out, your doctor can confirm whether you have IBS by using the validated and official IBS diagnostic criteria below (known as Rome IV criteria). To be diagnosed, you must fulfil all three criteria. Check the boxes that apply to you.

1. Recurrent tummy pain: On average, at least one day per week ☐

2. Pooping-related symptoms: Pain associated with two or more of the following:
   a) Pooping (i.e., pain improves or worsens when pooping) ☐
   b) A change in the frequency of your poop (i.e., pain is more common when your poops are more frequent or less frequent than usual) ☐
   c) A change in the appearance of your poop (i.e., pain is more common when your poops are softer or harder than usual) ☐

3. Persistent and chronic symptoms: Criteria 1 and 2 must have been present for the past three months and symptoms need to have started at least six months ago. ☐

If you don't meet all the criteria for IBS (for example, you have other gut symptoms, but not tummy pain), you may have another type of functional gut disorder (see page 147). Remember: It's important to see your doctor to rule out other conditions and to confirm a diagnosis of IBS—self-diagnosis can be risky business.

For those who do have IBS, what now? There are four subtypes of IBS. You may be pleasantly surprised to hear that determining your subtype is as simple as taking a peek at your poop (I told you it was informative stuff!). Using the Bristol Stool Scale from the Checking In with Your Poop assessment (page 25), you can determine your IBS subtype:

1. Think about your IBS in the last four weeks. On the days you had abnormal poops (i.e., type 1, 2, 6, or 7), how much of the time were they type 1 or 2?
   A) 25 percent or less of the time ☐
   B) More than 25 percent of the time ☐

2. Think about your IBS in the last four weeks. On the days you had abnormal poops, how much of the time were they type 6 or 7?
   C) 25 percent or less of the time ☐
   D) More than 25 percent of the time ☐

Classification of IBS Type:

If you checked

☐ **B AND C:** You have constipation-predominant IBS.

☐ **A AND D:** You have diarrhea-predominant IBS.

☐ **B AND D:** You have mixed IBS.

☐ **A AND C:** You have unsubtyped IBS.

As some of you may have already experienced, your subtype can change over time. One study found that around one in five people noticed a change in their subtype over a two-year period. You may also find it comforting to know that IBS was resolved in around half of the participants by two years. In practice, the number I see is much higher—particularly in those who work on the gut-brain axis—more on this in chapter 7.

DO YOU HAVE ANOTHER FUNCTIONAL GUT DISORDER?

Just as for IBS, there is no positive diagnostic test to confirm whether you have any of the other functional gut disorders; instead, they require that you rule out other conditions first. As a reference tool, I've included the criteria for three of the most common disorders that I see in my clinic. However, as with IBS, it's always best to discuss them with your doctor to ensure you're not missing anything.

The first criteria for all functional gut disorders is that the symptoms need to have begun at least six months ago (i.e., they're not just a short-term event) and that you've met the criteria for at least the last three months (i.e., the symptoms aren't resolving).

Check the boxes that apply to you.

Functional constipation

1. You don't meet the criteria for IBS. ☐

2. You experience two or more of the following:
   a) Straining during more than 25 percent of poops ☐
   b) Lumpy or hard poops (Bristol stool type 1 or 2) in more than 25 percent of poops ☐
   c) Feeling of incomplete evacuation (like you have not completely emptied your bowel) after more than 25 percent of poops ☐
   d) Feeling like something is blocking your poop from coming out in more than 25 percent of poops ☐
   e) Requiring physical strategies in more than 25 percent of poops (e.g., massage) ☐
   f) Fewer than three spontaneous poops per week. ☐

3. Loose poops are rarely present without the use of laxatives. ☐

Functional bloating/distention

1. You don't meet the criteria for a diagnosis of IBS or another functional gut disorder. ☐

2. Recurrent bloating and/or distention occurring, on average, at least one day a week; tummy bloating and/or distention predominates over other gut symptoms. ☐

Functional diarrhea

1. You don't meet the criteria for IBS. ☐

2. Loose or watery poops, without predominant tummy pain or bothersome bloating, occurring in more than 25 percent of poops. ☐

Source: Rome Foundation Working Group

In chapter 4, we discussed the dietary strategies for each of these predominant symptoms—check those out if you haven't already.

Changing Up Your Diet

Diet has revolutionized the management of IBS, with research demonstrating that the majority of people are able to effectively manage their symptoms by making changes to what they eat and drink. This makes sense, given that around 90 percent of people with IBS say that food triggers their symptoms. There are two main ways to tackle IBS symptoms through changes to your diet. The first-line approach has been shown to achieve impressive benefits in around 50 percent of IBS suffers. Better still, it's something you can start on your own. The second-line approach is a little more in-depth and involves restriction of a group of carbohydrates known as FODMAPs, many of which are prebiotics, followed by staged reintroductions.

Diet can be very effective in getting your symptoms under control, but it doesn't necessarily target the underlying cause of your IBS. As a result, if diet is the only change you make, when trigger foods are reintroduced, often the symptoms also return. I see diet not as the solution but as part of the solution. Diet changes typically begin to take effect anywhere from a few days to a few weeks, which gives your gut time to "rest" (as well as giving you some symptom-free sanity). It also allows time for the slower-acting complementary non-diet approaches to take effect, which I recommend you begin along with the changes in your diet. These non-diet approaches have been shown to target the disordered gut-brain communication, i.e., the underlying cause of IBS. They include sleep hygiene, mindfulness, gut-directed yoga, and breathing strategies, among others. We'll go through these in detail, along with exercises for you to try, in chapter 7.

Not everyone's IBS works in the same way, and research from my team suggests that some of these differences may explain why different people respond to different therapies. This reinforces the message that managing IBS is not a one-size-fits-all approach.

 Caution: *IBS dietary advice may trigger negative thinking patterns if you have a history of an eating disorder. Best to see a dietitian for support.*

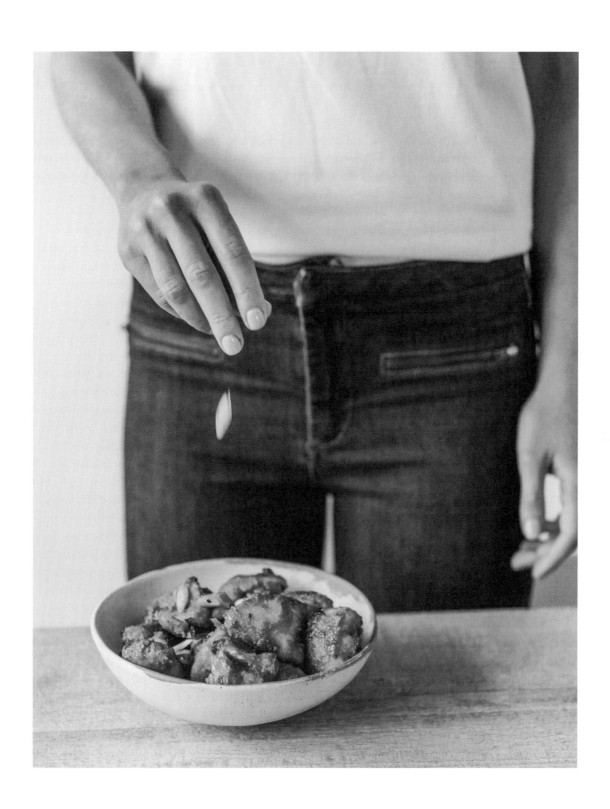

First-Line Diet Approach

It's both the way you eat and what you eat that can impact gut symptoms. This is because eating can affect gut movements, gut permeability (aka leakiness), stress hormones (yep, your diet can affect these, too!) and your GM. Despite this, most of us tend to focus all our attention on *what* we're eating and disregard *the way* we eat entirely.

Take one of my patients, Dan, a thirty-two-year-old lawyer. After Dan caught a stomach bug on holiday, his bowels were never the same. He suffered from altered bowel habits (some days diarrhea, others constipation), excessive bloating, tummy pain, and reflux for close to a year. Dan was convinced he was intolerant to a particular food but couldn't seem to pinpoint the culprit. He'd tried cutting out gluten, dairy, raw foods, cooked foods, acidic foods, and just about every other commonly victimized food you may read about online, but none of his attempts seemed to provide any benefit. In fact, he noticed that many of the restrictions made his symptoms worse. Dan was very diligent and came to our consultation with a typed list of all the foods he'd eaten in the previous week, along with a timeline of the symptoms he had experienced. I asked him to describe more about his actual eating patterns. He explained that he wasn't much of a morning person, so he had his first meal around noon, often on the run between meetings, and then wouldn't eat again until he got home, after 8:00 PM I probed a little further about how he ate his meals, and I could see he was a little confused. Why was I focusing on how he was eating rather than on the food list he had so diligently prepared? Noting Dan's confusion, I walked him through how digestion worked, explaining that the sheer act of filling the stomach leads to a release of communication molecules that stimulate the bowel and affect movement, among many other things. In some people, this can lead to discomfort soon after eating. Although a little hesitant, Dan agreed over the next four weeks to shift his focus from what he was eating to how he was eating. We agreed on two strategies: 1) to continue eating the same amount and type of food but to spread it across five eating times in a day; and 2) to eat only when sitting down and with technology switched off (phone, computer, and television). Four weeks later, the frequency of Dan's symptoms had halved and, after adding in stress-management techniques (including mindfulness, which we look at on page 189), he was back in control of his gut and his life within two months.

So what exactly does this first-line diet approach involve? It looks at both specific components of food known to stimulate the gut and your eating pattern. The first step will make good use of My Gut Diary from chapter 5.

Dietary Component	Main Sources and Considerations
ALCOHOL	All alcoholic drinks. Response is typically dose-dependent, meaning small amounts may be OK. Ciders, sweet wines, and rum may be worse because of their FODMAP content (see page 153). **RECOMMENDATION:** Drink no more than one standard drink a day (equivalent of around 12 ounces/350 ml low-strength beer, 5 ounces/150 ml wine, or 1.5 ounces/45 ml spirits). Or, if you're up for it, go without for the four-week trial.
CAFFEINE	See page 123. **RECOMMENDATION:** Limit to one caffeine-containing drink/food a day (e.g., 1 single shot coffee, 1 tea [50 to 100 mg caffeine per day]). Or, if you're up for it, go without for the four-week trial.
SPICY FOOD	Any dish containing chile peppers. **RECOMMENDATION:** Limit chile-containing meals.
FAT	Fried foods and fatty meats (e.g., fries, deep-fried chicken), pastries, cakes, chocolate, shortbread, pies, chips; full-fat cheese, cream, coconut milk. **RECOMMENDATION:** Limit large portions of high-fat foods, particularly those with limited nutritional value (i.e., high-fat fast food).
WATER	All liquids. **RECOMMENDATION:** Drink 50 to 70 ounces (1.5 to 2 L) of fluid per day (aim for mostly water).
DIETARY FIBER	Fruit, vegetables, whole grains, legumes, nuts, seeds, products fortified with fiber (such as inulin and oligofructose/fructo-oligosaccharide). **RECOMMENDATION:** Spread fiber intake evenly throughout the day. Aim for two pieces of fruit, five portions of vegetables, three portions of whole grains, and one or two portions of nuts/seeds/legumes each day. If your normal intake is greater than this, reduce for the four-week trial; if normal intake is lesser, gradually increase, as discussed on page 58.
FRUIT	Fresh, dried, juices, smoothies. **RECOMMENDATION:** No more than one piece of fruit per sitting (equivalent of 3 ounces/80 g fresh or 1 ounce/30 g dried) with up to three sittings across the day. Limit juices and smoothies; eat whole fruits.
POLYOLS	Sugar-free/low-calorie foods, chewing gum, and other food and drinks with added mannitol, maltitol, sorbitol, xylitol, or isomalt. **RECOMMENDATION:** Avoid all sweeteners ending in -ol (plus isomalt).

Follow the flow diagram below to determine the next step for you.

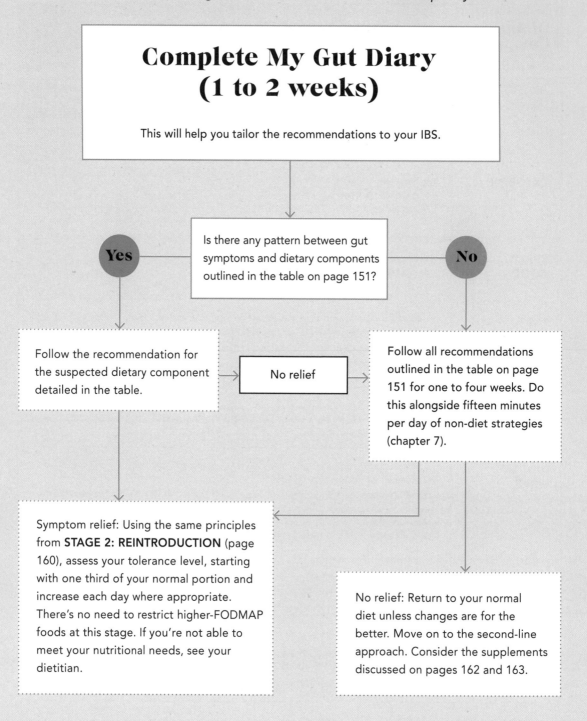

Complete My Gut Diary
(1 to 2 weeks)

This will help you tailor the recommendations to your IBS.

Yes

Is there any pattern between gut symptoms and dietary components outlined in the table on page 151?

No

Follow the recommendation for the suspected dietary component detailed in the table.

No relief

Follow all recommendations outlined in the table on page 151 for one to four weeks. Do this alongside fifteen minutes per day of non-diet strategies (chapter 7).

Symptom relief: Using the same principles from **STAGE 2: REINTRODUCTION** (page 160), assess your tolerance level, starting with one third of your normal portion and increase each day where appropriate. There's no need to restrict higher-FODMAP foods at this stage. If you're not able to meet your nutritional needs, see your dietitian.

No relief: Return to your normal diet unless changes are for the better. Move on to the second-line approach. Consider the supplements discussed on pages 162 and 163.

Second-Line Diet Approach

If it turns out your IBS is a little more stubborn, it's time to consider a low-FODMAP diet. The low-FODMAP diet was first developed by colleagues from Monash University in Australia and is backed by a body of good-quality trials, with success seen in around 70 percent of people.

What Are FODMAPs?

FODMAPs are a group of carbohydrates found in a wide range of foods that are poorly absorbed in the small intestine. At the risk of getting too sciencey on you, *FODMAP* stands for fermentable oligosaccharides, disaccharides, monosaccharides, and polyols, which are the scientific names given to groups of carbohydrates based on their chemical structure. The table below helps break things down. Within each of these carbohydrate groups, there are specific types that are restricted during the initial stage of the low-FODMAP diet.

Carbohydrate Groups	Carbohydrates Restricted Short-Term	Key Dietary Sources
OLIGOSACCHARIDES	Fructans (Fructo-oligosaccharides [FOS] & inulin) Galacto-oligosaccharides (GOS)	Wheat, rye, specific fruits and vegetables (e.g., onion and garlic), and added prebiotics Legumes, such as kidney beans
DISACCHARIDES	Lactose	Specific dairy products (e.g., milk from animals)
MONOSACCHARIDES	Excess fructose*	Specific fruits, juices, honey, high-fructose corn syrup, some flavored waters
POLYOLS	Including mannitol and sorbitol	Specific fruits and vegetables Some low-calorie sweeteners, particularly those in sugar-free gums, mints, and low-calorie products

Remember: Not all foods that contain fructose are restricted. As we discussed on page 122, many fruits contain enough glucose to help with the fructose absorption or, in the case of the theater analogy, the glucose opens up that second viewing room.

How Does It Work?

Unlike other carbohydrates (such as glucose), FODMAPs aren't completely absorbed in the small intestine. Instead, they end up in the large intestine, which results in two things:

- **EXCESS FLUID:** The undigested carbohydrates (FODMAPs) can draw fluid from the body into the intestine, effectively dumping a load of extra fluid and increasing the pressure on the intestinal wall. This may also overwhelm the large intestine's ability to absorb the fluid, which can result in mushy, loose poops. Others may find that, although the start of their poop is hard and constipation-like (acting like a plug), the end of their poop may actually be loose.

- **FERMENTATION:** Yes, this is the GM food frenzy. As we touched on above, the FODMAPs entering the large intestine are rapidly eaten (fermented) by our GM. As a result, a burst of gas is released. Although this also occurs in people without IBS, in those with visceral hypersensitivity, the stretching of the intestine activates the nerves around the intestine, triggering pain signals to the brain and activating the tummy-distention reflex discussed on page 96.

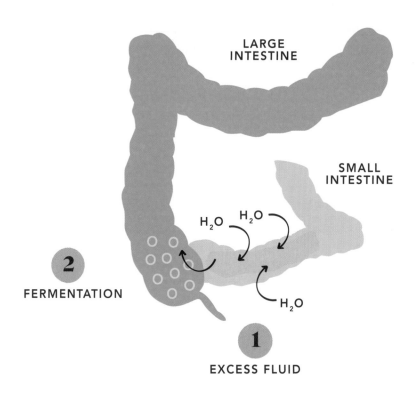

LARGE
INTESTINE

SMALL
INTESTINE

H_2O H_2O

2
FERMENTATION

H_2O

1

EXCESS FLUID

What Does It Involve?

A low-FODMAP diet consists of three stages, with the end goal being a personalized, modified FODMAP diet. You may read the stages below and feel slightly overwhelmed by the complexity of the diet. That's exactly why guidelines recommend that you embark on the low-FODMAP diet only with the support of a FODMAP-trained dietitian or healthcare professional.

1

RESTRICTION STAGE: This is what people commonly refer to as the low-FODMAP diet, in that you restrict all high-FODMAP foods. It can help to think of this stage as giving your sensitive intestine some downtime. Guidance from a dietitian is critical at this stage, in order to tailor the diet to your nutrient needs. If you don't respond to the diet after six weeks, revert to your usual diet and consider other therapies. Make sure you do go back to including FODMAPs in your diet, because many FODMAPs are actually beneficial for your gut microbes in the long term, as we discuss in the following pages.

2

REINTRODUCTION STAGE: After following the restriction stage for two to six weeks (depending on how quickly your symptoms improve), reintroduce each of the different FODMAPs one at a time, in portions guided by your dietitian. This stage will help you identify which FODMAPs you're most sensitive to and the amount of offending FODMAPs you can tolerate without triggering symptoms. This can take several months to complete.

3

PERSONALIZATION STAGE: This is also known as the modified or personalized FODMAP diet (your long-term diet) and is the end product of stages 1 and 2. This diet is tailored to your personal FODMAP tolerance. Stage 3 not only gives your diet flexibility and variation, a key factor in achieving long-term compliance, but also keeps your GM happy and, above all, improves your food-related quality of life. Keep in mind that tolerance typically improves over time with the continuation of those gut-brain-axis strategies, which we discuss in chapter 7. For this reason, retesting foods that you previously didn't tolerate is a good idea.

Principles Worth Knowing

- **A LOW-FODMAP DIET IS NOT FODMAP-FREE.** The diet categorizes food as "high" or "low" FODMAP, based on a cut-off level of FODMAPs per portion. This means that even low-FODMAP foods may contain some FODMAPs.

- **IT'S ALL ABOUT THE SIZE OF THE PORTION.** A high-FODMAP food may be low-FODMAP if the portion size is reduced. An example is wheat pasta. One cup of cooked wheat pasta is considered high FODMAP, whereas half a cup is considered low FODMAP.

- **LACTOSE IS A "CONDITIONAL" FODMAP.** If you've gone through the 3R Method on page 126 and are confident that you're not lactose intolerant, then you don't need to restrict lactose in your low-FODMAP diet. With that in mind, even if you are lactose intolerant, you can still tolerate small amounts of lactose, as discussed on page 140. This is why the restriction stage allows some cow's milk (up to ¼ cup/60 ml per sitting) and other dairy products that contain small amounts of lactose, such as hard cheeses (see page 135).

- **FODMAPS ARE CARBOHYDRATES.** It's helpful to remember that foods free of carbohydrates, such as meats, seafood, egg, fats, and oils, are naturally free of FODMAPs (unless of course they've been marinated or use carbohydrate fillers/substitutes).

- **A LOW-FODMAP DIET IS NOT GLUTEN-FREE.** It is easy to get confused, because a low-FODMAP diet also restricts gluten-containing grains such as wheat, barley, and rye. The difference is that a low-FODMAP diet restricts the large amounts of fructans found in these grains, rather than the gluten. The diet only restricts significant amounts of these grains, and lesser amounts can still be included, such as small amounts of wheat used in sauces. In contrast, a gluten-free diet restricts even trace amounts of these grains.

- **FODMAPS ARE NOT INHERENTLY BAD.** Many FODMAPs, such as fructans, are actually prebiotic, meaning they feed your good gut bacteria! This is why it's super important to reintroduce FODMAPs into your diet after a maximum of eight weeks of restriction. Why restrict them at all? The research shows that those with visceral hypersensitivity typically benefit from a short break (think of it as gut rest) while you work on that dysfunctional gut-brain axis with strategies discussed in chapter 7.

Mile-High IBS

Do your symptoms get worse on airplanes? There is some science behind this phenomenon. Air trapped inside your gut expands as the airplane climbs, thanks to the change in atmospheric pressure (this also explains why your ears pop and your water bottle or packages of food expand). What might be only a little bit of gas at ground level can expand in the sky, putting extra pressure on your intestines. This happens to everyone, but because those with IBS typically have a more sensitive intestine, this extra pressure can lead to feelings of bloating and pain. The solution? Cutting back on higher-FODMAP foods (see page 159) twenty-four to forty-eight hours before you fly may help.

Real-World Approach

I once tried to follow the low-FODMAP diet, not because I had IBS but because I wanted to experience it from my patients' perspective. I failed miserably! In the first week, I made a ton of mistakes; the second week, I ate the same meal four nights in a row because work was crazy busy and I hadn't planned ahead; and by the third week, I was craving my Fudgy Black Bean Brownies (page 279) so badly that I pulled the plug. This experience taught me two things: First, my patients' symptoms must be pretty bad for them to be motivated enough to stick to this diet for up to six weeks; and second, this diet requires a lifestyle that is ideal in terms of time and space to cook from scratch. This got me thinking: Do all my patients really need to go the whole way to see benefits? It turns out that, *no*, they don't—a simplified low-FODMAP diet, or "FODMAP-lite" approach, restricting only a subset of high-FODMAP foods, is enough for many people with IBS to get control over their IBS.

> Take, for example, twenty-one-year-old Toni. Toni had just moved out of home for college and was sharing an apartment with five others. Having been diagnosed with IBS in high school and trying first-line strategies with little benefit, Toni was keen to do whatever it took to get her symptoms under control before her final exams. But it was clear that a low-FODMAP diet was not going to be appropriate for Toni's current lifestyle. In fact, it might have actually contributed to Toni's stress-induced symptoms due to the difficulty of following it. When I reviewed Toni's diet, I could see she was consuming large amounts of FODMAPs and was a good candidate for the FODMAP-lite approach (alongside mindfulness strategies). Within two weeks on the modified diet, her symptoms had improved, and by week four, she described her symptoms as "completely under control." Using the FODMAP-lite approach, Toni was able to move swiftly through the next two stages. She identified her breakfast smoothie, large amounts of legumes, date-based energy balls, and low-calorie sweets as her main triggers. To manage these, she turned her breakfast smoothie into whole foods—oats, fruit, and yogurt; reduced her portion of legumes at each sitting to her tolerated amount; and started making her own energy balls without the dates. As for the daily fifteen minutes of mindfulness, Toni found it had the added benefit of improving her concentration, so she stuck with it long-term.

If your IBS doesn't respond to the first-line diet approach and you don't have access to a FODMAP-trained health care professional, the FODMAP-lite approach might be a helpful place to start. But don't just jump straight into it (this is the mistake I made with the full diet). Spend time becoming familiar with the higher-FODMAP foods and planning your meals without them. This will help you get the most out of the diet and minimize the burden and duration needed to see a benefit.

Select Higher-FODMAP Foods to Limit	Key Dietary Sources
VEGETABLES	Artichokes, asparagus, broccoli, brussels sprouts, cabbage, cauliflower, chicory root, garlic, leeks, mushrooms, onions, scallions (white part), peas.	Carrots, chives, cucumber, eggplant, ginger, green beans, kale, peppers, potatoes, spinach, squash, tomatoes, zucchini, pickled garlic and onion.
FRUIT	Apples, apricots, blackberries, boysenberries, cherries, dates, figs, mango, nectarines, peaches, pears, persimmons, plums, prunes, watermelon, fruit juice (more than ⅓ cup plus 1 tablespoon/100 ml), foods/drinks with added fruit concentrate.	Blueberries, clementines, honeydew melon, grapes, kiwis, lemons, limes, oranges, passion fruit, pineapple, raspberries, rhubarb, strawberries. Maximum of one piece of any fruit per sitting (equivalent of 3 ounces/80 g fresh, 1 ounce/30 g dried, ⅓ cup plus 1 tablespoon/100 ml juice), with a maximum of three sittings throughout the day.
PROTEIN SOURCES	Legumes (e.g., baked beans, chickpeas, kidney beans, soybeans), pistachios, and cashews.	All fresh meats (e.g., chicken, fish, lamb), eggs, firm tofu, walnuts, Brazil nuts. Canned and (thoroughly) rinsed legumes contain fewer FODMAPs compared to those boiled from dry. Therefore, small portions (¼ cup per sitting), particularly of canned chickpeas, butter beans, and adzuki beans, are better tolerated; ½ cup of canned lentils is considered low FODMAP.
GRAINS	Large amounts of wheat-based foods.	Quinoa, rice, buckwheat, millet, oats, polenta. Keep to ½ cup (125 g) of cooked wheat, barley, or rye-based foods (including couscous and semolina) or 1 slice of bread per sitting, with up to three throughout the day.
OTHER	Agave, honey, high-fructose corn syrup, fructose, and low-calorie sweeteners ending in -ol (see page 151). Added inulin, fructo-oligosaccharide, galacto-oligosaccharide in some yogurts and cereals.	Maple syrup, table sugar (sucrose), glucose.

*This is not a comprehensive list. It's here to give you inspiration. Include all other foods that are not listed in the "higher-FODMAP" column in your diet. Remember, this is a modified version, not the full low-FODMAP diet.

FODMAP-Lite Approach

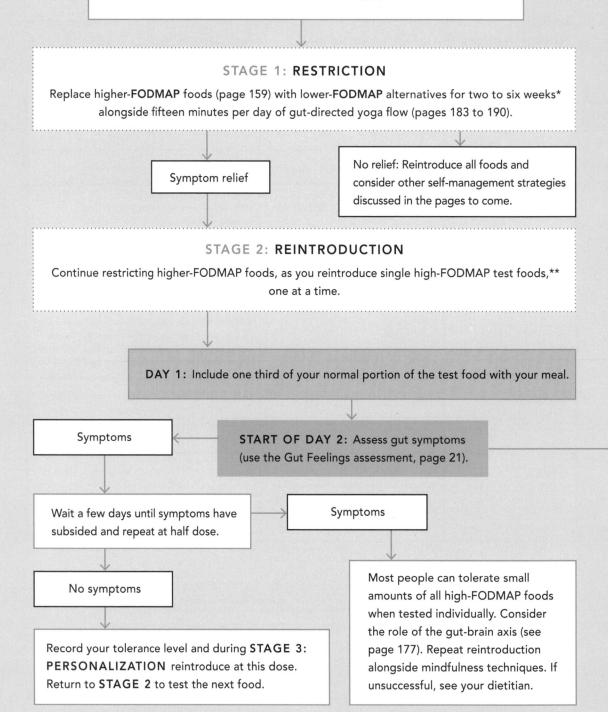

STAGE 1: RESTRICTION

Replace higher-**FODMAP** foods (page 159) with lower-**FODMAP** alternatives for two to six weeks* alongside fifteen minutes per day of gut-directed yoga flow (pages 183 to 190).

Symptom relief

No relief: Reintroduce all foods and consider other self-management strategies discussed in the pages to come.

STAGE 2: REINTRODUCTION

Continue restricting higher-FODMAP foods, as you reintroduce single high-FODMAP test foods,** one at a time.

DAY 1: Include one third of your normal portion of the test food with your meal.

START OF DAY 2: Assess gut symptoms (use the Gut Feelings assessment, page 21).

Symptoms

Wait a few days until symptoms have subsided and repeat at half dose.

Symptoms

No symptoms

Record your tolerance level and during **STAGE 3: PERSONALIZATION** reintroduce at this dose. Return to **STAGE 2** to test the next food.

Most people can tolerate small amounts of all high-FODMAP foods when tested individually. Consider the role of the gut-brain axis (see page 177). Repeat reintroduction alongside mindfulness techniques. If unsuccessful, see your dietitian.

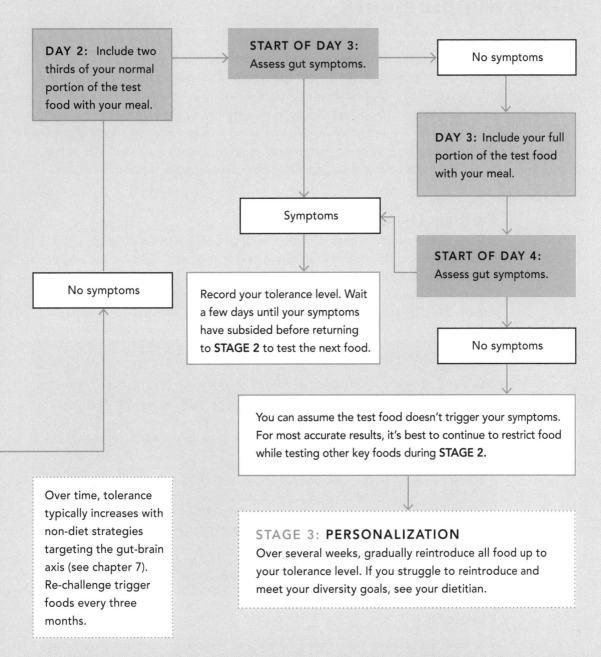

DAY 2: Include two thirds of your normal portion of the test food with your meal.

START OF DAY 3: Assess gut symptoms.

No symptoms

DAY 3: Include your full portion of the test food with your meal.

Symptoms

START OF DAY 4: Assess gut symptoms.

No symptoms

No symptoms

Record your tolerance level. Wait a few days until your symptoms have subsided before returning to **STAGE 2** to test the next food.

You can assume the test food doesn't trigger your symptoms. For most accurate results, it's best to continue to restrict food while testing other key foods during **STAGE 2**.

Over time, tolerance typically increases with non-diet strategies targeting the gut-brain axis (see chapter 7). Re-challenge trigger foods every three months.

STAGE 3: **PERSONALIZATION**
Over several weeks, gradually reintroduce all food up to your tolerance level. If you struggle to reintroduce and meet your diversity goals, see your dietitian.

* *Ensure you are maintaining adequate amounts of fruit, vegetables, and whole grains.*

** *TEST FOODS: Choose suspected trigger foods from higher-FODMAP foods (page 153).*

Fiber Supplements

Fiber in IBS can be a little confusing. Not only is the amount important—either too much or too little in your diet can trigger symptoms—but the type of fiber also matters. My research group is currently undertaking a multinational trial on IBS to look at whether we can combine the benefits of various fibers (both normalizing poop and improving the happiness of the GM) without inducing symptoms. We aim to achieve this by using a mixed-fiber supplement (one of the fiber types includes psyllium; more on that in what follows). I won't bore you with all the intricacies; instead, let's focus on the most promising fiber supplements currently available.

Psyllium (Ispaghula)

This unique fiber has dual functionality, thickening up loose poops but at the same time softening hard poops. Therefore, it's thought to benefit all types of IBS by normalizing poop output. It may also improve other symptoms, such as bloating and incomplete evacuation. On its own, however, psyllium is unlikely to resolve all your IBS symptoms, so if you are interested in supplements, I recommend you use it in combination with other strategies.

Psyllium Prescription

Start with 1½ teaspoons per day and see how things go. You may like to increase it to 1 tablespoon per day in the second week if needed, gradually increasing up to 3 tablespoons per day if useful and tolerated. If there's no improvement after one month, stop. If your gut is extra-sensitive, you may like to start with 1 teaspoon per day. The practical tips:

- *It's available from most health food stores.*
- *It forms a thick gel when mixed with cold water (similar to what happens in your gut), so it's best combined with oatmeal or warm soup. I often add to my DIY Granola, too (page 225). Use ½ cup plus 2 tablespoons (150 ml) of fluid per tablespoon.*
- *Check in with your doctor if you need to continue taking it for over six months.*
- *Like many fibers, psyllium can decrease your appetite. If you are underweight, it may be best to stick to the half dose and continue to monitor your weight. If your weight decreases, stop and discuss with your dietitian.*

Flaxseed

In terms of food sources, there's some evidence for flaxseed in constipation-predominant IBS (IBS-C). If you want to give it a go, I recommend that you start with 1½ teaspoons per day and gradually increase up to 2 tablespoons per day over four weeks, as needed and tolerated. Sprinkle some on your breakfast, yogurt, salads, or soups. Be sure to include an extra ½ cup plus 2 tablespoons (150 ml) fluid per 1 tablespoon of flaxseeds. Check out the high-flaxseed Cheesy Vegan Crackers on page 269.

Peppermint Oil

Unlike many other herbal supplements, the benefits of peppermint oil in IBS have been rigorously studied and are backed by quality science (and a heap of anecdotes from my patients, too). Peppermint oil is an antispasmodic, which means it works by relaxing a tense intestine, which is common in IBS. As a result, peppermint oil has been shown to significantly reduce tummy pain.[42] It may also help relieve tummy bloating and excess wind by supporting more efficient gas transport.

What about peppermint tea? The studies showing the benefits of peppermint oil have only used coated peppermint-oil capsules.[43] Why does the coating matter? It stops the oil from being digested in the stomach, ensuring it make its way into the small intestine, where the peppermint works its magic. That's not to say that drinking peppermint tea is pointless: If you find it helps, do what works for you.

The Practical Stuff

If you're interested in giving peppermint oil a try, studies recommend taking one capsule (providing 0.2 ml or 180 to 225 mg of peppermint oil) up to three times a day, thirty minutes to an hour before a meal. It's generally best to take on an empty stomach and away from antacids. Most studies have used specific peppermint oil capsules, which are widely available from health stores or online. In terms of safety (because anything in a high dose is always worth checking), peppermint capsules have been shown to be well tolerated, but long-term studies haven't been conducted, so you might like to consider tapering down after four weeks. Anything beyond two months is worth discussing with your healthcare team.

Managing Stubborn Tummy Pain

If diet and supplements don't relieve your tummy pain, and natural remedies, like applying a heat pack to the painful site, don't work, talk to your doctor about medications that can help. These include antispasmodics such as hyoscine butylbromide (e.g., Buscopan), which can be handy to keep in your bag if you're prone to unpredictable IBS-related cramping episodes. For long-term pain, there's a group of medications known as central neuromodulators that have proven effective by targeting the gut-brain pain pathway. Interestingly, these central modulators are a type of antidepressant, which are prescribed for IBS at much lower doses.

Small Intestinal Bacterial Overgrowth

Commonly referred to as SIBO, small intestinal bacterial overgrowth is character-ized by an increased number of microbes invading the small intestine. The small intestine is much more sensitive than the large intestine, so it doesn't fare well when having to accommodate these extra microbial guests (and their fermenting feasts). As a consequence, they can interfere with the small intestine's normal func-tion, causing IBS-like symptoms such as tummy pain, bloating, excess flatulence, and diarrhea.

It's still early in terms of our understanding of SIBO, but it is thought that it may overlap with or account for a subset of IBS. Breath tests are commonly used in practice to support diagnosis. However, there are considerable limitations with breath tests, and therefore interpretation of results should be guided by a special-ist gut doctor (gastroenterologist) or trained healthcare professional.

Disappointingly, there's limited research into the dietary management of SIBO, although a low-FODMAP diet is likely to reduce gut symptoms. This is because the low-FODMAP diet decreases the amount of fermentable food available in the lower end of the small intestine where the overgrowth occurs, essentially starving the overgrown microbe community. The standard therapy for SIBO is antibiotic treat-ment. Research suggests that combining the antibiotic with a special fiber known as hydrolyzed guar gum, which you can buy online or from health food stores, may have a greater benefit compared to using the antibiotic alone (one study showed an 85 percent success rate with the combination, compared to 62 percent with antibi-otics alone).[44] Another small study demonstrated that combining the antibiotic with a probiotic also enhanced the effectiveness.[45] Nonetheless, it's worth keeping in mind that the relapse rates post-antibiotic are disappointingly high. This is because antibiotics only treat the symptoms and not the underlying cause of the overgrowth. Discuss ways to prevent relapse of SIBO with your gut doctor.

Digestive Enzymes

Specific enzymes such as alpha-galactosidase can help break down the FODMAP (called GOS) found in legumes and some nuts (such as cashews and pistachios). Research from Dr. Christopher Tuck and colleagues demonstrated that, compared to placebo, alpha-galactosidase significantly improved tolerance to foods high in GOS in IBS patients (who reported symptoms from eating foods high in GOS).[46] The dose of the enzyme appeared to be important, with benefit seen using 300 GALU (galactosidic units), half given immediately before the GOS-loaded meal (e.g, a bowl of baked beans) and the other half during the meal.

Now, because I find that most of my patients are able to reintroduce foods high in GOS over time, I don't often need to recommend these enzymes. Nonetheless, there have been some cases where legumes are a favorite food or people are traveling to countries where legumes are a staple food, in which case they've come in really handy to improve people's food-related quality of life. The enzymes are available online or from selected health food stores. Similarly, if you find lactose is a trigger, you can consider lactase enzymes.

What about other digestive enzymes? I wouldn't bother at this stage, as there is insufficient evidence for broad-spectrum digestive enzymes, such as those available over the counter, unless you have pancreatic insufficiency, which is rather rare and should only be diagnosed by your doctor. In such cases, over-the-counter digestive enzymes will not be enough; instead, you will be prescribed enzyme supplements at a much higher strength.

Could It Be a Leaky Gut?

Triggers of a Leaky Gut ·

As I alluded to on page 20, leaky gut is not a black-and-white "syndrome." In fact, the tight junctions (remember, they're like the bouncer on the door outside a club) between the cells that make up the wall of our intestine open and close all the time in response to a variety of things. This includes diet (e.g., a high-fat meal), exercise (e.g., strenuous endurance running), medication (e.g., some painkillers) and, perhaps not surprisingly, stress. The role of stress was shown in a clinical trial where they measured the gut leakiness in people before and after public speaking. The study found that those who were more nervous and stressed were the ones whose gut became leaky.[47] Now, before you start freaking out (and trigger further stress-induced leakiness), rest assured that these factors tend to have only a short-term effect on the tight junctions and don't seem to cause any major issues. In some diseases, exposure to proteins (e.g., eating gluten if you have celiac disease) has a more sustained and severe effect on the tight junctions and therefore the leakiness of the gut. But if you have celiac disease and strictly avoid gluten in your diet, the tight junctions do their job and the leaky gut resolves. This explains why a sustained leaky gut is considered more a symptom of an underlying disease rather than the cause of disease.

How Do We Diagnose It?

There are several ways to measure how leaky your gut wall is. One way we measure it in clinical trials involves drinking different types of sugars and measuring the sugar concentrations in urine over several hours. Some sugars are too big to be absorbed across a normal intestine, which means that, if they're found in the urine, it's likely because the wall of the intestine is leaky and is letting things through that it shouldn't. But before you go out and spend your hard-earned cash on measuring your gut leakiness, think to yourself: What's the purpose? What's the benefit? I personally believe that, outside of research, for most people, there's not a lot to gain by measuring your gut leakiness. Why? Not only will the results likely differ from day to day, but both human and animal studies have shown that a leaky gut alone is insufficient to initiate disease. Therefore, the current scientific consensus is that a leaky gut is indeed a symptom rather than a cause of disease. What's even more important is that, despite research investigating both diet and novel drug therapies to target gut leakiness, to date, none have proven effective. So, in short, yes, you can measure it, but it's not going to change or inform how you manage your symptoms—not just yet, anyway.

Where to from Here?

As the science currently stands, it is unlikely that a sustained leaky gut is the root of your health problems—but instead it may be a symptom of one. With this in mind, it makes more sense to focus on the underlying cause of your gut symptoms, such as stress, rather than the symptoms, that is, a leaky gut. That said, the dietary recommendations discussed in chapter 3 may also support the health of those tight junctions. Specifically, several polyphenols and short-chain fatty acids (discussed on page 54) derived from plant-based foods are known to support the tight junctions, at least in animal studies.

Period Problems

As some of you know all too well, IBS symptoms can get worse leading up to and/or during menstruation. This is related to fluctuating hormones that affect not only your uterus but also your gut, affecting motility, sensitivity, and levels of inflammation. If your periods are particularly painful or heavy, however, it's worth visiting your doctor to be assessed for endometriosis, a condition that affects as many as one in ten people with uteruses. Despite many overlaps with IBS, some of the red flags for endometriosis include difficulty conceiving, painful sex, and heavy periods.

Maybe It's Not IBS

If you've got diarrhea-predominant IBS (IBS-D) (see the assessment on page 146), pay particular attention to whether your symptoms are worse after high-fat meals. If you see a pattern and notice that your diarrhea improves on a low-fat diet, it's worth discussing the possibility of bile acid diarrhea (BAD) with your doctor. Why? As I mentioned on page 16, bile acids are released to help our body absorb fat, and 95 percent of bile acids are normally reabsorbed in the small intestine, but, in some cases, they're not. Instead, the bile acids enter the large intestine, causing havoc and resulting in diarrhea. Research suggests that as many as 30 percent of people with IBS-D may actually have BAD, which means that malabsorption of the bile acids in the intestine is causing the diarrhea, not IBS. If this is the case, there are different management strategies, including both medication and dietary approaches, which are best discussed with your doctor and dietitian, respectively.

When Self-Management Is Not Enough

If your symptoms are still getting the better of you after you've tried the strategies detailed in this chapter, it's time to call in the gut experts. I know this can be frustrating, but remember, we've only touched on the basics here; there are plenty of other strategies your doctor, dietitian, and gastroenterologist have up their sleeves. If you're feeling alone on your journey, most countries have IBS support groups that you can tap into—they have been life-changing for many of my patients. (Check out aboutibs.org.)

CHAPTER 7

Beyond Diet:
Sleep, Stress, and Exercise

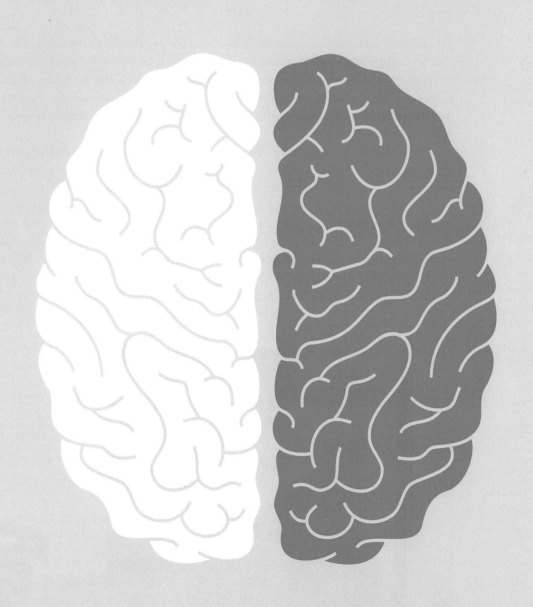

Beyond Diet

Let's explore what else you can do to take your budding relationship with your gut to the next level. Outside of diet, there are three areas I see as being key for good gut health: sleep, stress, and exercise. Their importance for overall health is clearly nothing new, but what is new is our understanding of how they affect our gut microbiota (GM). If we really want to harness the full potential of our gut health, we also need to get these three main areas in check.

Advice around "sleeping more" and "stressing less" has become redundant: We all know we should be doing it, yet too few of us are. Life happens—I totally get it. This is why I want to share with you the tools, the exercises, and the strategies, and help you fit them in around everything else going on in your life. For those of you who are thinking, *I don't have time for this—I'm just going to stick with diet*, I hear you, but here's the thing: You can have the "ultimate" gut-boosting diet, but if you're not sleeping right or your stress levels are through the roof, your gut health will likely pay the price. Just as they say that no amount of exercise can outdo a bad diet, no amount of gut-healthy eating can outdo a disastrous lifestyle. Balance really is the key to your GM's heart.

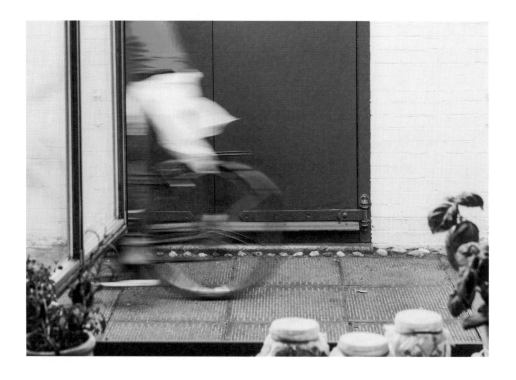

One of my patients, forty-three-year-old Emma, experienced firsthand the importance of balance. Emma was a single mom, juggling full-time work and raising two young kids. She was considered quite the superwoman among her friends.

Over two months, we worked together to get Emma to a place where she had good control of her symptoms through diet, apart from the occasional episode. After some troubleshooting, we identified poor sleep and stress as two of her key triggers. To target these areas, Emma and I developed a fifteen-minute program of strategies (many of which are covered in this chapter) as a preventative measure, to help Emma cope when these unavoidable circumstances arose. Three months later, when I saw her again, I could tell from the look on her face that something had happened. Emma recounted her worst episode yet. She'd been at work when the tummy pain began; within an hour, it had become so crippling that she'd had to swallow her pride and ask her colleague to take her to the emergency room and her neighbor to collect her kids from school.

How had this happened? Emma explained that she'd had a very hectic month and, between a promotion at work and looking after the kids, her fifteen-minute program had dropped off her schedule. Reflecting back, it was clear to her that by not allowing herself those fifteen minutes each day, it ended up costing her over three days in downtime (that's over 2,000 minutes!) at the expense of both her family and work.

Emma's case is an extreme example of how not taking a few moments each day to look after yourself could end up costing you much more in the long run. I think there's something we can all learn from Emma's experience: Are you taking at least fifteen minutes a day to focus on your health and happiness?

For each of these non-diet "heavy hitters," we'll go through a range of practical strategies and exercises that I've seen make a meaningful impact on people's lives. It's a good idea to record the ones that resonate with you in your Gut-Health Action Plan on page 210. Throughout this chapter, keep in mind that something is better than nothing. Even if you only manage to add in a small change, you'll still be one step ahead of where you were yesterday.

Sleep

One of the most underrated resources at your disposal to support optimal (gut) health is sleep. Like our human cells, our GM has a circadian rhythm (a body clock), so disturbed sleep can also affect its natural rhythm, as we touched on in chapter 2. Studies have shown that sleep deprivation can affect our GM after just two days. Sleep deprivation can also increase inflammation and stress hormones in your body, which may explain why not getting enough sleep is linked with gut symptoms, particularly in people with irritable bowel syndrome (IBS).

Work by my colleagues at King's College London has shown that lack of sleep can also affect how much you eat.[48] And it's not by a nominal amount either—the review study suggested that partial sleep deprivation increased daily intake by the caloric equivalent of four slices of bread. As you may have experienced yourself—I know I have—this extra food tended not to be the quality high-fiber stuff: The study showed that sleep-deprived people reached for more high-fat, lower-protein foods, keeping all the nutrition to themselves and leaving none for their poor GM (who, don't forget, have also been sleep-deprived).

When you haven't had enough sleep, you are also more susceptible to getting sick. One study, which used identical twins to control for genetics, found that sleep deprivation was linked with lower immunity[49] (remember: 70 percent of our immune cells live in the gut).

Before we move on to looking at the practical strategies to help boost your pillow time, let's think about your sleep quality. How refreshed do you feel most days?

Assessment: LET'S TALK ABOUT SLEEP

The following questions relate to your usual sleep habits during the past month. I know sleeping habits are not always the same, but try to think about your average sleep when completing this assessment.

1. What is your usual?

    BEDTIME _____ GETTING UP TIME _____ = _____ HOURS SPENT IN BED

2. How long (in minutes) does it usually take you to fall asleep?

Fewer than 15 minutes (0 points)	15 to 30 minutes (1 point)	31 to 60 minutes (2 points)	More than 60 minutes (3 points)

3. How many hours of actual sleep do you get at night? (This may be different from the number of hours you spent in bed.)

Fewer than 5 hours (3 points)	5 to less than 6 hours (2 points)	6 to 7 hours (1 point)	More than 7 hours (0 points)

4. What is your sleep efficacy? This is your hours spent sleeping (answer from question 3) divided by hours spent in bed (answer from question 1) =

0.85 or higher (0 points)	0.84 to 0.75 (1 point)	0.74 to 0.65 (2 points)	0.64 or less (3 points)

5. How would you rate your sleep quality overall?

Very bad (3 points)	Fairly bad (2 points)	Fairly good (1 point)	Very good (0 points)

6. How often have you taken medicine to help you sleep (prescribed or over-the-counter)?

None (0 points)	Less than once per week (1 point)	1 to 2 times per week (2 points)	3 or more times per week (3 points)

7. How often have you had trouble staying awake while driving, eating meals, or engaging in social activity?

Never (0 points)	Less than once per week (1 point)	1 to 2 times per week (2 points)	3 or more times per week (3 points)

Your score : _____

SCORE INTERPRETATION

Very good sleep quality   Very poor sleep quality

0 points ————————————————➤ **18 points**

Adapted from the Pittsburgh Sleep Quality Index. Visit sleep.pitt.edu for the full version.

One in three adults don't get enough good-quality sleep[50]—how did yours rate? If your sleep quality is on the lower end, rest assured, it's certainly not a life sentence. And what about your immune system? Are you frequently catching the flu, or do you struggle to shake an infection?

Assessment: HOW GOOD IS YOUR IMMUNITY?

As we touched on in chapter 1, our gut microbiota (GM) plays a key role in training and supporting our immune system. So with that in mind, let's have a look at how your immune system is faring.

Think about how often you've had these symptoms and conditions over the past year. If you haven't heard of some of the conditions, then it's unlikely you've had them, which is a good thing, so don't worry. Circle one number per row.

		Never	Once or twice	Occasionally	Regularly	Frequently
1.	Sore throat	4	3	2	1	0
2.	Headaches	4	3	2	1	0
3.	Flu	4	3	2	1	0
4.	Runny nose	4	3	2	1	0
5.	Coughing	4	3	2	1	0
6.	Cold sores	4	3	2	1	0
7.	Boils	4	3	2	1	0
8.	Mild fevers	4	3	2	1	0
9.	Warts	4	3	2	1	0
10.	Pneumonia (lung infection)	4	3	2	1	0
11.	Bronchitis (lung infection)	4	3	2	1	0
12.	Sinusitis (swelling of the sinuses)	4	3	2	1	0
13.	Sudden high fever	4	3	2	1	0
14.	Ear infection	4	3	2	1	0
15.	Episodes of diarrhea (not related to IBS or other chronic conditions)	4	3	2	1	0
16.	Meningitis (acute inflammation around the brain)	4	3	2	1	0
17.	Eye infection	4	3	2	1	0
18.	Sepsis (infection in the blood)	4	3	2	1	0
19.	Slow-healing injury	4	3	2	1	0

Source: Gastroenterology[51]

Your score : _____

How does your immune strength rate? There are many things at play when it comes to our immune system—some things outside of our control, like genetics, and others within our control, such as how well fed and rested our GM is. If your immunity seems to be on the lower end of the scale, working to improve and nurture your GM with diet (check out the recipes in chapter 9) and sleep (more in this chapter) really can help.

Improving your sleep can be achieved by making small changes to your lifestyle. Colleagues Dr. Haya Al Khatib and Dr. Wendy Hall proved this in a trial where, using simple sleep-hygiene strategies (detailed in the following), they were able to significantly improve not just participants' sleep duration but their sleep quality, too.[52] They also showed the benefit of improved sleep on diet. In fact, compared to the control group (who maintained their usual sleeping pattern), those who applied the sleep strategies reduced their intake of added sugars by two teaspoons per day—which is pretty impressive, given that diet wasn't the focus.

Sleep-Hygiene Protocol

What does sleep hygiene *actually mean? It's a phrase that describes the habits you can put in place to optimize the length and quality of your sleep. The result? You feel much more well rested and begin to reap the effects, including benefits to your immunity, diet, and other areas of your well-being, such as mood.*

STEP 1: Identify four habits from the sleep-hygiene checklist that are relevant and realistic targets for your lifestyle.

STEP 2: Implement your chosen strategies for a minimum of four weeks.

STEP 3: After four weeks, reassess your sleep quality using the sleep quality assessment (Let's Talk About Sleep; page 172).

STEP 4: Reevaluate your selected strategies and adjust as needed, keeping in mind that it typically takes nine weeks of daily practice to form a habit (or sixty-six days, to be exact, according to research from University College London).[53] If you have persistent sleeplessness, talk to your doctor or a sleep expert for support.

Sleep-Hygiene Checklist

1. A REGULAR ROUTINE: Maintaining the same sleep time and wake time every day (give or take thirty minutes) can help your body's and GM's clock to function at their best.

2. BEDROOM ENVIRONMENT: Make your bedroom a relaxing environment that you use only for sleep (and bonding with your partner). To do this, keep your bedroom:

   - **Dark:** Make sure to keep your bedroom only dimly lit at night by using dimmers or lamps with low-wattage bulbs. Consider investing in some thick curtains (or an eye mask).

   - **Tidy and quiet:** Clutter and noise can distract your mind from relaxing. Try some earplugs, if you need them.

   - **At a slightly cool temperature (around 65°F/18°C):** Your body's temperature starts to drop as you fall deeper into your slumber, so it helps not to get too warm while you sleep.

3. MORNING LIGHT: Light is how your environment communicates with your body clock. Exposing your face to natural light first thing in the morning helps support and reset it. Whether it's going for a five-minute walk outside, or doing some stretching in your backyard, waking your body with natural light is a really refreshing way to start your day.

4. TECHNOLOGY (INCLUDING TVS, LAPTOPS, PHONES, AND OTHER GADGETS): Blue light from backlit screens is particularly disruptive to your body's clock. It counteracts your ability to produce melatonin, which is an important hormone for sleep. Avoid these in the hours before bedtime. If you must use them, consider installing blue light filter apps on your device.

5. NAPPING: Avoid excessive napping (more than twenty minutes) during the day. If you nap, you may not feel tired enough to fall asleep at night.

6. AVOID CAFFEINE AND STIMULANTS: These oppose your body's attempts to wind down before bedtime. It's best to limit them after 3:00 PM.

7. FULLNESS/HUNGER: Going to bed too full or too hungry can disrupt your sleep. Depending on the size of your meal, waiting at least two to three hours before bed can be helpful. Similarly, if you are too hungry, you may be too distracted to fall asleep and may wake up through the night wanting a snack.

8. A BEDTIME ROUTINE TO HELP YOU UNWIND:

   - Have a warm bath (not too hot) to relax you and help your body reach a temperature that is ideal for rest.

   - Relaxation exercises, such as gentle stretching, can help your muscles to relax.

   - Listen to music that calms you, or use a guided smartphone meditation app to help calm your thoughts.

   - Reading a book in dim light is a great alternative to being on your phone or laptop in the bedroom.

9. SCHEDULE "WORRY TIME": We often struggle to fall asleep if we're worrying. It may sound counterintuitive, but allowing yourself some time during your day to worry and write down all your thoughts and to-do lists can give you the mental space to relax before bed.

Stress: Rewiring the Gut-Brain Axis

It's easy to get caught up in trying to "perfect" your diet and forget that our brain has a big impact on our gut, too. If you're a little skeptical, as I first was, let me share the research with you. Several trials have compared, head to head, the effectiveness of the standard diet for IBS, a low-FODMAP diet (page 153), and non-diet approaches that target the gut-brain axis.[54] The non-diet approaches included cognitive behavioral therapy (CBT), relaxation techniques, hypnotherapy, and yoga. Strikingly, several trials showed that the non-diet interventions improved gut symptoms to the same degree as the dietary interventions. Just think about that for a moment: One intervention solely targeted trigger foods and the other just the gut-brain axis, and both had the same outcome. (The non-diet approaches do take a little longer to take effect, so stick with them for at least twelve weeks.)

Rather than removing foods that can trigger the gut, the non-diet approaches work on the underlying cause: The dysfunction between the gut and brain via the vagus nerve. The vagus nerve is the part of the nervous system that we likened to a mobile phone in chapter 2, acting as a communication highway that connects our brain and our gut (and almost every other organ in between). This nerve plays a crucial role in breathing, heart rate, immune response, and digestion. It's also part of the parasympathetic system (PNS, the rest-and-digest control center), which, when activated, has the effect of settling the sympathetic system (SNS, the fight-or-flight control center).

I used to rely on two ways to assess the impact of the gut-brain axis on my patients' symptoms. First, I'd ask them to rate their general day-to-day stress levels, and second, I'd get them to consider whether their symptoms improved when they were on vacation. From this quick assessment, I would determine how much of a priority it was to focus on stress, but after meeting twenty-four-year-old Kelly, I realized assessing stress was not that straightforward. Kelly had been diagnosed with IBS and had been referred to me for dietary advice by her gastroenterologist. I went through my standard assessment, and Kelly had a below-average stress score and no change to gut symptoms on vacation. She appeared to be a good candidate for the low-FODMAP diet. At our follow-up review, as I'd expected, Kelly's symptoms had resolved, but what I didn't expect was the way they'd resolved. Hint: Diet had nothing to do with it.

Kelly had been following the low-FODMAP diet for two weeks before she went away for a friend's wedding. At that stage, Kelly hadn't noticed much improvement in her symptoms but was committed to following the diet for at least four weeks, despite the challenges of doing so while on vacation. Within a few days of being away, she noticed her symptoms were starting to improve, despite not being as strict with the diet as she'd intended. By day five, Kelly described herself as feeling like a new woman; after years of battling with her symptoms, it seemed they had disappeared. The eczema across her chest had also started to clear up. A few days later, Kelly returned from the wedding and continued to follow the diet. But, within days, her symptoms returned with a vengeance. "As defeating as it was," she said, "I'm glad it happened. It was the wake-up call I needed to realize I was unconsciously battling stress."

Kelly had an easygoing boss, a loving partner, and no money issues—she felt she didn't have the right to be stressed, so she suppressed any feelings of it. Like many of us, Kelly always jam-packed her holidays with activities and never really switched off for more than a day. "This time," Kelly reflected, "every element was organized for me. I just had to show up. I slept in most days and lay by the pool. There was bad internet, so I didn't bother with my phone—it was the first time in years that I'd truly disconnected."

With this new level of awareness, Kelly had begun to see a psychologist and, within three weeks of therapy, was starting to get that new-woman vibe back. Diet-wise, we reintroduced all high-FODMAP foods and moved toward the Gut Health on a Plate principles (pages 78 to 79).

Kelly's story is a familiar one. Modern life is so busy that many of us underestimate how stressed we really are. In fact, in many cultures, being stressed has become the new norm and being busy a badge of honor. While we may be used to it, the signs of this unconscious stress often present in other ways such as troubled sleep, unstable mood, and gut issues.

Assessment: IS STRESS GETTING THE BEST OF YOU?

Although it's normal and often beneficial for everyone to get a little stressed from time to time, if it's frequent or debilitating when it does strike, your (gut) health is likely paying the price. Even if you don't think you're stressed, it's worth checking.

The questions in this tool ask you about your feelings and thoughts during the last month. In each case, circle how often you felt or thought a certain way. Like the happiness questionnaire, some of the questions are phrased negatively, and others positively, so take your time reading through them.

	Never	Almost never	Sometimes	Fairly often	Very often
1. How often have you been upset because of something that happened unexpectedly?	0	1	2	3	4
2. How often have you felt that you were unable to control the important things in your life?	0	1	2	3	4
3. How often have you felt nervous and "stressed"?	0	1	2	3	4
4. How often have you felt confident about your ability to handle your personal problems?	4	3	2	1	0
5. How often have you felt that things were going your way?	4	3	2	1	0
6. How often have you found that you could not cope with all the things that you had to do?	0	1	2	3	4
7. How often have you been able to control irritations in your life?	4	3	2	1	0
8. How often have you felt that you were on top of things?	4	3	2	1	0
9. How often have you been angered because of things that were outside of your control?	0	1	2	3	4
10. How often have you felt difficulties were piling up so high you could not overcome them?	0	1	2	3	4

Source: Journal of Health and Social Behavior[55]

Your score : _____

SCORE INTERPRETATION

Very relaxed   Super-stressed

0 points ━━━━━━━━━━━━━━━━━━━━━━▶ 40 points

If you are toward the more stressed end of the scale, take comfort in the fact that there is plenty you can do to help get those scores down, starting with the exercises on pages 180 to 190.

If your score is above 30, it might be worth talking to someone about it. If you don't feel like you're able to talk to your family or friends (give them a try first, though; they may surprise you), ask your doctor about community services that may help you.

The Strategies

Many of us, including myself, have at some stage fallen for the idea that it's good to be constantly on the go. But our brains and bodies are not made for this; they become fatigued, and this raises stress levels, decreases resilience, and affects our GM. Rest is as important as activity for our physical, mental, and gut health. Gut-brain expert psychologist Kimberly Wilson recommends two of her favorite exercises to help target your gut-brain axis that you can try out in the comfort of your own home.

EXERCISE 1: THE DO-NOTHING EXERCISE

This exercise is essentially scheduled inactivity. Many stressed people find this one really challenging, as they worry about being unproductive or "lazy." Sometimes, underlying this is a feeling that, if we stop, we won't have the energy to start again. This is a good clue to how tired and stressed we really feel.

"Do nothing" is exactly that. Pick a point in the day where you do absolutely nothing. Ideally, it's best to lie down so that there isn't even any physical stimulation. With that in mind, many people find it best to do this at the end of the working day, when they get home. It's particularly useful before having a meal.

Place a notepad and pen beside you (you won't need them until the end). Set a timer for ten minutes (if using your phone, be sure to switch it to silent). Lie down on your back; you can have your knees up or down, whichever is more comfortable. Rest your hands on your tummy or by your side. Take one or two deep breaths to settle yourself, and then just notice what happens. Consider the questions below. Try to stay with these experiences and, at the end of the ten minutes, write down your observations.

This exercise can give you really good insight into your attitudes toward yourself. Is it good to be busy? Do you imagine that someone else seeing you have a rest would call you lazy? Seeing these ideas written down in black and white can help you to challenge them in exercise 2.

Try this exercise once in the first week and slowly build up to at least five times a week, particularly on your busiest days.

- **HOW DOES YOUR BODY FEEL?** Are your shoulders or neck tight? Is your breathing deep or shallow?

- **WHAT MOOD ARE YOU IN?** Are you tired? Relaxed? Anxious? Do you feel guilty for "wasting time"?

- **WHAT'S HAPPENING IN YOUR MIND?** Are you thinking about your to-do list? Are you counting down the minutes before you can get up again? Maybe other thoughts or ideas come to mind.

EXERCISE 2: CHALLENGING JUDGMENTAL THOUGHTS (COGNITIVE BEHAVIORAL THERAPY)

The do-nothing exercise often throws light on our unconscious mental habits. Typically, we hold ourselves to much higher standards than we do others. We are much more critical of ourselves than we would be of a friend, or even a stranger, in the same situation. This constant internal pressure (as well as external demands) is a major driver of stress and poor coping. Recognizing and managing stress is dependent on our ability to be compassionate to ourselves, to treat ourselves like we would our best friend. I know it can be an odd concept for many, but trust me: It's worth thinking about.

One way to start challenging judgmental thoughts about yourself is to imagine you are hearing your own story from someone else. If a friend told you they were pushing themselves nonstop and never giving themselves a break, what would you say? Would you tell them to just suck it up, that they should be able to keep up with the pace, or would you say, "Wow, it sounds like you're under a lot of pressure"? Would you be curious about why they were being so hard on themselves? Write down the kinder and more balanced things you would say to a friend. Then, when those critical, pressurizing thoughts come up, try directing the more supportive thoughts to yourself. It's important to begin with something that feels manageable, so start by challenging just one critical thought that you've experienced. Once that positive challenge becomes automatic, you can move on to another critical thought.

Sometimes, critical thoughts and beliefs are deeply entrenched, and it can be helpful to see a cognitive behavioral therapist, who can help support you in understanding where those thoughts may have come from and how to challenge them.

Depending on how you scored on the stress assessment (see page 178), it might be a good idea to try to stick to at least one of these exercises for twelve weeks. I know sticking with things is easier said than done. To help, check out my top habit-forming tips on page 206.

Yoga

Yoga is a practice of the mind-body (and, I'm convinced, GM, too) that originated thousands of years ago. Coming from a science background, I thought yoga was a little too hippie-dippie for me for a long time. However, after putting my preconceived judgements aside and experiencing it for myself, I realized that not only did it improve my own focus, but it was also underpinned by several scientific principles. In fact, a systematic review (remember, that's the collection of evidence from multiple trials) has suggested that yoga practice may actually decrease inflammation markers in our blood, meaning there are tangible benefits of yoga for our whole body. Another review has shown benefits in people with high blood pressure. I've got some anecdotes from my clinic, too, where several patients have had their doctors reduce (and some even stop) their blood pressure medication after three months of practicing a daily yoga flow, including the breathing exercises on pages 184 and 185. In terms of gut disorders, it has been a game changer for the long-term management of many of my patients, too.

Yoga can relax a distressed gut in several ways. Not only does the breathing activate the PNS, that "rest and digest" system, but yoga also teaches you how to embrace new and often uncomfortable feelings in your body through improved control of your breathing as you explore various positions. This valuable technique can be applied to episodes of tummy pain or other gut symptoms; instead of resisting, which creates greater anxiety and stress, yoga teaches you to breathe through the discomfort. The physical movements, flowing between gentle compression and stretching, also send pulses along your intestine. This can help calm overall stimulation of the muscles and nerves and release any trapped gas (so if you get the urge, let it out!). And the cherry on the top: Most yoga sequences also end with relaxation, which you can think of as "resetting" the gut-brain axis.

As we touched on, one trial found that yoga had equal benefits to a low-FODMAP diet, with over 80 percent of participants reporting significant improvement in their IBS symptoms.[56] This research sparked my partnership with yoga teacher Richie Norton to develop a yoga sequence specifically for people with gut distress. Inspired by the postures used in the trial, we've developed a fifteen-minute sequence to make it a manageable daily addition to your morning or evening routine. Try it out and, for real results, stick with it for at least twelve weeks, as the participants did in the trial.

Gut-Directed Yoga Flow

The flow consists of four parts, all equally important: the warm-up, the breath, the moves, and the calm. All help manage the physical and psychological symptoms of stress. Many of my patients who suffer from IBS-related tummy pain have found implementing this practice, as soon as they feel an episode coming on, hugely beneficial in preventing the symptoms from escalating.

The Warm-Up

1. FIND A QUIET PLACE WHERE YOU CAN SIT WITHOUT BEING DISTURBED. You can sit on the floor, on a cushion, or on a chair—wherever you feel most comfortable sitting upright, with a straight back to prevent squashing your belly.

2. START TO BRING AWARENESS TO YOUR BREATHING, taking deep breaths in through your nose, then pausing for a few moments before gently releasing with a long, slow exhale, again through the nose. As you breathe in, feel the coolness of the air in your nostrils and its warmth as you breathe out.

3. ONCE YOU'VE FOUND A STEADY, CALMING BREATHING RHYTHM, begin to slowly loosen and mobilize the neck, shoulders, and back with some gentle rolling movements, being mindful not to rush this.

 Caution: *If you have issues with low or fluctuating blood pressure, it's best to discuss the breathing exercises with your doctor first.*

The Breath

1. Sitting upright, connect to a deeper "belly breath" (see below), making the inhale full and the exhale relaxed for ten breaths. If you've got some extra time on your hands, give the "humming bee breath" a try. Each style of breathing can relax you in different ways, so you might like to alternate between them.

2. If you are new to yoga and these breathing practices, it may feel more comfortable to start off by breathing in through your nose and out through your mouth. Over time, you can move to breathing in and out through your nose and see whether it makes a difference to how calm you feel.

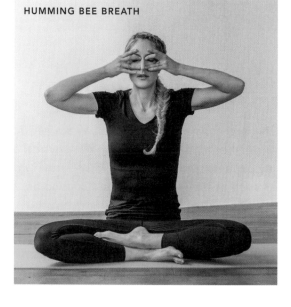

HUMMING BEE BREATH

BELLY BREATH
(Diaphragmatic Breathing)

1. Place one hand on your chest and the other on your belly. Start by taking a relaxed, deep breath in through your nose. Take note of which hand moves more, before gently releasing the air out through your nose (or mouth, if you prefer).

2. With your next breath in, allow your belly and rib cage to expand out, feeling your bottom hand rise while the hand on your chest remains still. This is a diaphragmatic breath. When you do this in reverse and the hand on your chest moves more, you are chest breathing. Chest breathing is designed for great exertion, which we subconsciously tend to activate in stressful situations. Making a conscious note to switch to diaphragmatic breathing in these situations can have a powerful calming effect.

HUMMING BEE BREATH
(*Bhramari pranayama*)

1. Sitting upright, with your eyes closed, raise your elbows to shoulder height and close your ears with your thumbs. Place your index finger above each eyebrow. Cover your eyelids with your middle fingers and place your ring finger beside the flare of each nostril (as pictured above).

2. Take a slow, deep breath to fill your lungs. Partially close your nostrils and breathe out through your nose, making a humming sound. Continue the humming for four seconds. Repeat five to ten times, extending the humming duration as you begin to feel more comfortable with it.*

This is a great tool to use when you feel stress arise during the day. Whether it's a missed train, bad emails, or lost keys . . . it's a game changer.

The Moves (Asanas)

For those new to yoga, stick with the foundation flow detailed below. If you're more experienced, you may like to add in the advanced positions noted with a double asterisk (**) to extend your flow. Hold each pose for at least three slow breaths.

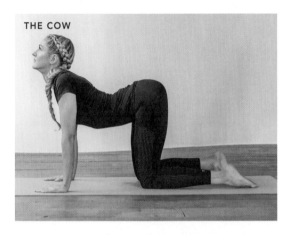

THE COW

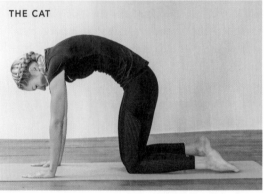

THE CAT

CAT-COW (*Chakravakasana*)

Start on all fours with your shoulders stacked over your hands and your knees positioned below your hips. Begin with some light movements side to side, forward and backward.

- **COW** (*Bitilasana*)
  Inhale, tilting your tailbone up, lifting your head and opening the chest, gazing slightly upward. Be careful not to compress your neck.

- **CAT** (*Marjaryasana*)
  With your exhale, tilt your chin to the chest, and push away from the ground, opening your shoulders and back. (Tip: Visualize pulling your belly button into your spine.)

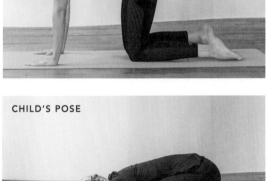

CHILD'S POSE

CHILD'S POSE (*Balasana*)

Return to your deep breaths (in and out through your nose), open out the knees and hips and ease yourself back, pushing from the hands until you are sitting over your heels. Let your forehead gently rest on the ground, letting your arms settle comfortably in front of you. Rest and breathe into the belly.

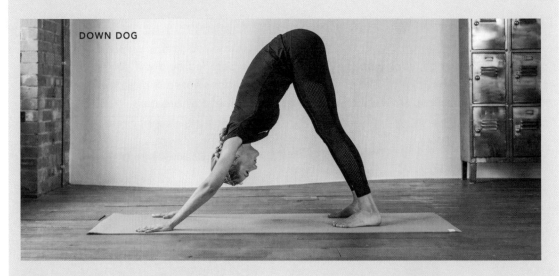

DOWN DOG

OPTIONAL: DOWNWARD-FACING DOG (*Adho mukha svanasana*)**

Move back onto all fours. Rolling your toes under, lift your knees off the ground, pushing your chest back toward your thighs. Try straightening your legs as much as your flexibility will allow, and push your heels down to the ground (don't worry if they don't touch). Breathe through the gentle stretch that radiates along the back of your legs, continuing to move your chest toward your thighs, maximizing the stretch across the back of your shoulders.

OPTIONAL: STANDING FORWARD BEND (*Uttanasana*)**

From downward-facing dog, walk your hands back toward your feet. Let your shoulders hang heavy over your feet. Slide your hands up along your legs, slowly bringing your chest parallel with the floor. Hold for one breath before moving to a full standing position, extending your arms wide, then drawing them in to meet above your head. Slowly lower your hands down the center of your body, resting them in front of your chest bone in the prayer position.

Inhale, folding forward back into downward-facing dog.

BABY COBRA (*Ardha bhujangasana*)

Lie flat on your belly with your forearms flat and your hands in line with your shoulders. Take a breath in and, on the exhale, gently push away from the floor, keeping contact along the arms. (Tip: Engage your leg muscles and lightly contract your glutes, i.e., your butt muscles.) Open up the front of your chest and belly. Relax back down and repeat.

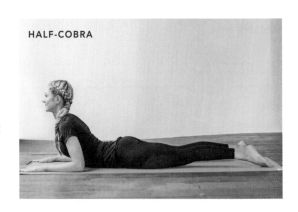

HALF-COBRA

OPTIONAL: LOCUST POSE (*Salabhasana*)**

Lie flat on your belly with your arms down by your side, palms planted on the floor. Gently contract your lower back muscles and raise your chest and arms. Hold for two breaths before relaxing back down. Next, contract your glutes and lift your legs off the ground, pushing your pelvic bone into the floor. Relax down. Combine both movements together.

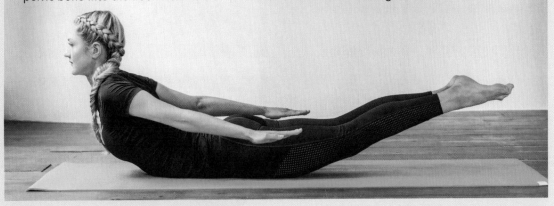

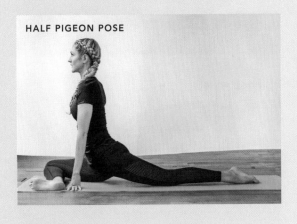

HALF PIGEON POSE

OPTIONAL: HALF PIGEON POSE (*Ardha kapotasana*)**

Bring your right leg forward in between your hands and rest your knee next to your right hand, with the sole of your foot facing your left hand (depending on your flexibility, your knee may be at anywhere from a 15- to a 90-degree angle). Gently lower your body weight evenly into both hips, keeping them straight, and extend your left leg back.

As you inhale, lengthen through the upper body and, as you exhale, sink a little deeper into your hips, pressing your left leg back into the floor and evening out the hips. Repeat on the other side.

SAGE TWIST (*Marichyasana*)

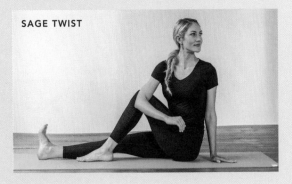

SAGE TWIST

Sit upright with your legs extended in front of you. Bend your left knee and hug it toward your chest. Place your left hand behind you for support as your right elbow moves to your left knee, lightly twisting the body. Repeat the twist on the other side.

CROCODILE TWIST (*Supta matsyendrasana*)

Lying on your back, tuck both knees into your chest and gently rock side to side and back and forth, lightly massaging your back. Release the legs down before bringing your right leg across your body. Look to your opposite shoulder, hold, and breathe. Repeat on the other side.

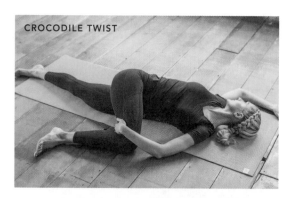
CROCODILE TWIST

HAPPY BABY POSE (*Ananda balasana*)

Inhale, bringing both knees into your chest. Bring your arms through the insides of your knees and hold onto the outside edge of each foot. Gently pull your knees down toward your underarms. Visualize pressing your tailbone down into the floor as you press your heels up, keeping them flat, as if you were standing on the ceiling. Press the shoulders and the back of your neck down into the floor, aiming to flatten your whole spine. Rock across your back, left to right. Smile like a happy baby.

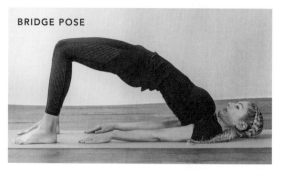
HAPPY BABY

BRIDGE POSE (*Setu bandhasana*)

Lying on your back with your knees bent, push off the floor with your feet, lifting the hips, tightening your glutes to support your back, and keeping your chin tucked into your chest. Breathe.

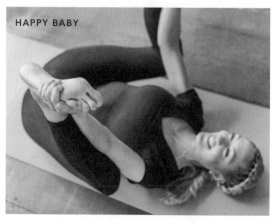
BRIDGE POSE

CORPSE POSE (*Savasana*)

Lower your back flat on the floor, bring your knees to your chest, and rock side to side, forward and back. Then lay your legs out straight, allowing your feet to fall out to the side (open hips). Close your eyes, be still, and breathe.

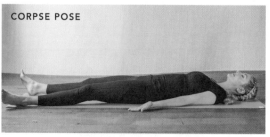
CORPSE POSE

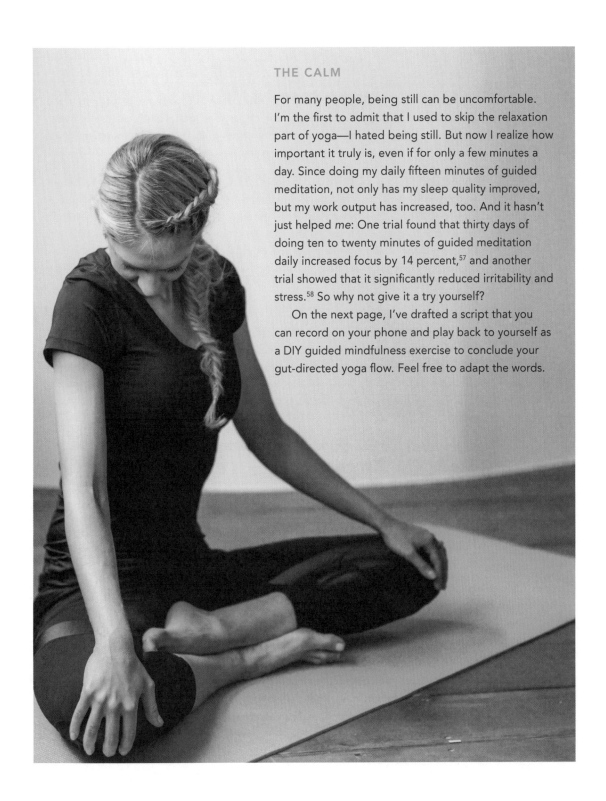

THE CALM

For many people, being still can be uncomfortable. I'm the first to admit that I used to skip the relaxation part of yoga—I hated being still. But now I realize how important it truly is, even if for only a few minutes a day. Since doing my daily fifteen minutes of guided meditation, not only has my sleep quality improved, but my work output has increased, too. And it hasn't just helped *me*: One trial found that thirty days of doing ten to twenty minutes of guided meditation daily increased focus by 14 percent,[57] and another trial showed that it significantly reduced irritability and stress.[58] So why not give it a try yourself?

On the next page, I've drafted a script that you can record on your phone and play back to yourself as a DIY guided mindfulness exercise to conclude your gut-directed yoga flow. Feel free to adapt the words.

The Script

- **TAKE A FEW MOMENTS TO GET COMFORTABLE,** whether it's staying in the corpse pose or sitting up with a straight back, cross-legged. Gently close your eyes. Begin by bringing your attention into a deep, slow belly breath, in through your nose and out freely through your mouth. Repeat for five breaths.

- **BEGIN TO MOVE YOUR FOCUS INTO THE REST OF YOUR BODY.** Feel the weight of your body on the ground underneath you, the contact of your arms against your body. Slowly scan down your body, starting from the top of your head. Without buying into or analyzing them, softly note any physical feelings or emotions that might be present, just observing them, like you would traffic passing you by. Continue down to your belly. Feel your stomach muscles relaxing as you visualize them melting away any tension with each breath. Continue scanning down your body, all the way to your toes.

- **LET YOUR MIND REST BACK ON THE PHYSICAL SENSATION OF THE BREATH,** noticing the rhythm and how each breath is a little different from the last. Continue for ten long, slow breaths, maintaining the curiosity as you sit with each unique breath. It's completely normal for your mind to wander off; when it does, gently acknowledge the thought or feeling before bringing your attention back to your breath.

- **BRING YOUR FOCUS BACK INTO THE BODY AND YOUR SURROUNDINGS,** noting the contact between your legs and the ground and the air on your skin. Note any background sounds or smells. Take a few breaths here. With your final deep breath, feel the oxygen filling your body and a deeper sense of relaxation as you exhale out, this time through your nose.

- **IN YOUR OWN TIME,** and only when you're ready, slowly open your eyes. Before you get up, take a moment to appreciate how it feels to have given yourself these fifteen minutes to reconnect with your mind and your body (and your GM, too). Hope to see you back here tomorrow.

> If you find this part of the flow beneficial, you might like to try a meditation app, such as Headspace or Calm, which offer a range of mindfulness exercises to suit different needs. Whatever you choose, the most important thing is to make this a daily habit. For those new to mindfulness, I get that, initially, the breathing and stillness can feel a little uncomfortable. But, with time, I can assure you that your mind and body will start to crave the clarity that yoga can bring.

Exercise: Move Your Body

We all know exercise is good for us, but the idea that it also benefits our GM may be the extra incentive we need to get moving. While most of the current research comes from observational and animal studies, more is emerging in actual humans (go figure) suggesting that the link between exercise and a diverse GM is independent of diet. This means that it's not just because people who exercise tend to eat more healthily. The study also found that the benefit relied on sustained exercise, so hitting the exercise hard for a few weeks and then burning out and stopping is not going to do your GM much good in the long term.[59]

When it comes to the type of exercise, funnily enough, your GM likes whatever you do (or perhaps they've wired us to like whatever they do). As long as you're moving your body often, getting your heart rate up for at least thirty minutes most days, you'll be satisfying everyone's needs.

Assessment : HOW ACTIVE ARE YOU?

So how are your fitness levels? Over the past three months, how many minutes per week did you spend doing:

1) Moderate-level exercise (where you could talk, but not sing, during the activity)?

Less than 30 mins (0 points)	30 to 89 mins (1 point)	90 to 149 mins (2 points)
150 to 209 mins (3 points)	210 to 269 mins (4 points)	270+ mins (5 points)

2) Vigorous exercise (where you couldn't say more than a few words without pausing for a breath)?

Less than 15 mins (0 points)	15 to 44 mins (1 point)	45 to 74 mins (2 points)	75 to 104 mins (3 points)
105 to 134 mins (4 points)	135 to 164 mins (5 points)	165+ mins (6 points)	

Your score : _____

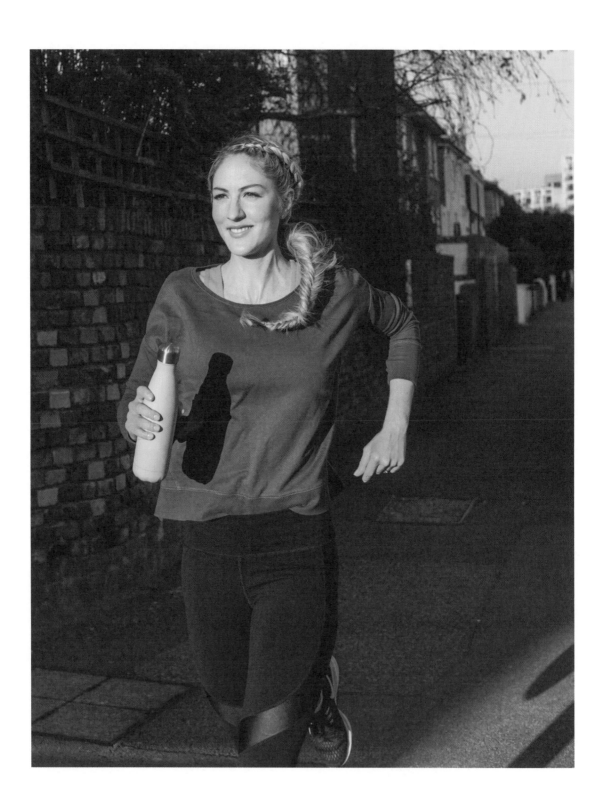

A score of 3 points is in line with national guidelines (that is, for heart fitness; it's also suggested that you do strength exercises at least two days a week—anything from lifting weights, weight-bearing exercises like yoga, or even heavy gardening such as digging; anything that works all your major muscles counts). Need more convincing? One study demonstrated that a change from 0 to 6 points (from sedentary to 180 minutes of vigorous exercise a week) resulted in an improvement in participants' GM composition and function, i.e., which bacteria were there and what they did, independent of diet.[60]

Exercise is not just about training for heart fitness and perfecting our running technique; there's another side to it, a more targeted type—have you ever considered your bowel fitness or pooping technique?

This unconventional type of fitness is not to be dismissed—it has revolutionized the way in which many gut symptoms are managed, particularly constipation, urgency, and incontinence (when you can't hold your poop back). What about if you don't have any symptoms? Is it still relevant? Absolutely. Maintaining your bowel fitness is also helpful in the prevention of issues as we age and our pooping muscles weaken. For those who plan to conceive one day, it's even more crucial, with as many as 50 percent of moms who give birth vaginally having issues with this.

Bowel-Training Exercises

With the help of bowel-training expert Ellie Bradshaw and pelvic health physiotherapist Lucy Allen, we've got some basics to get your bowel fit.

Correct Pooping Position

Did you know that the human body was designed to poop in the squatting position? It's a fact seemingly overlooked by the masterminds behind the sitting toilet. It may also be no coincidence that countries with sitting toilets (much of the Western world) have an increased risk of pooping issues. But don't worry: You don't need to let your elevated toilet define you. Here's how you can get your pooping position just right.

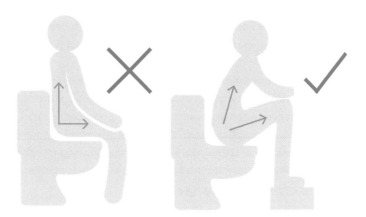

1. WHEN SITTING ON THE TOILET, ENSURE YOUR KNEES ARE SLIGHTLY HIGHER THAN YOUR HIPS. For this, you can utilize an old phone book or shoe box, or invest in a foot stool to place under your feet.

2. LEANING FORWARD, PROP YOUR ELBOWS ON TOP OF YOUR KNEES.

3. ENSURE YOUR SPINE IS STRAIGHT AND BULGE OUT YOUR TUMMY (everything below the belly button).

4. RELAX AND LOWER YOUR SHOULDERS.

There you have it: the toilet position that straightens out the bottom of the intestine and the anus, the exit point, allowing for a smooth departure.

How to Be a Good Pooper

Pooping is rather like dancing: Everyone can do it, but for some of us it requires a little more effort and concentration to master the moves. How good a pooper you are is not just down to your inherent ability to coordinate the muscles but also determined by learned behaviors from as far back as your toilet-training days.

For those struggling with constipation or incomplete evacuation (where you don't feel like you've emptied your bowels properly), follow the steps below to help ensure the appropriate coordination of your pooping muscles.

1. ONCE IN THE CORRECT POOPING POSITION, move your hands around the sides of your waist and cough. Feel your waist widen. These are the muscles to use when pooping.

2. MAKE YOURSELF AS WIDE AS POSSIBLE BY BROADENING AT THE WAIST and bulging out the lower tummy. Bear down to create pressure and propulsion for two to three seconds, as if you are trying to force out gas. Relax a while, then repeat. Do this a few times both to initiate and complete emptying.

Many people strain from their chest, which is counterproductive. Why? This can cause tightening of your outer pooping sphincter and pelvic floor muscles, blocking the "exit" pathway.

If you're suffering from constipation and feel like you'd benefit from more training, talk to your doctor about seeing a biofeedback specialist nurse like Ellie.

Strengthening the Pelvic Floor

The pelvic floor is a sheet of muscles, likened to a trampoline, extending from your tailbone to your pubic bone (back to front) and from one side of your butt bones to the other (side to side). This muscle is not only crucial for keeping our intestine (and other organs such as the bladder) in place, preventing prolapses, but it's also important for maintaining bowel and urine continence. Essentially, it keeps us in control of our urges and prevents any "leaks," whether we're doing jumping jacks in the gym or stranded without a toilet in sight.

A weak pelvic floor is very common—a third of all women experience a problem with their pelvic floor over their lifetime.[61] Getting on top of it early will help you beat this statistic. If this isn't enough of an incentive, it also improves your sex life.

How to Strengthen Your Pelvic Floor Muscles

1. TO CONTRACT YOUR PELVIC FLOOR MUSCLES, start by tightening your back passage (anal sphincter), as if to stop gas from coming out. Then extend the contraction, lifting up and forward to your pubic bone, as if you are also trying to stop the flow of urine. This is your pelvic floor muscles contracted.

2. ACTIVATE AND HOLD YOUR PELVIC FLOOR MUSCLES FOR UP TO TEN SECONDS. If you can't feel the muscle still squeezing by the ten-second mark, it means your pelvic floor is a little weak. If so, try starting with a shorter hold.

3. REPEAT STEP 1 AS MANY TIMES AS YOU CAN, relaxing for five to ten seconds in between each squeeze, until you feel the muscles starting to get tired. This may be between five and a maximum of fifteen repetitions.

4. NOW TRY QUICK "SNAPS," tightening up the muscle back to front quickly, relaxing for a few seconds, then repeating. Make sure that, in between each squeeze or snap, you fully relax the muscle, breathing naturally as you are holding. If you feel your butt clenching, your eyebrows rising, or that you've forgotten to breathe, you may be trying too hard (happens to the best of us). Aim for ten to fifteen snaps each time.

If you can complete at least five of the ten-second holds, doing these exercises once a day is enough to maintain strength and function. For those with weaker pelvic floors (less than five holds), try to do these exercises three times a day. I know it sounds like a lot, but the good thing about them is that they can essentially be done anywhere. Waiting for the train, cooking dinner, even when sitting in a meeting—no one will ever know.

Caution: *Not all pelvic floor problems are fixed by strengthening them. If you have any of the problems below, it's best to get the advice of a physical therapist, as sometimes the pelvic floor muscles can get too tight or sensitive, causing difficulty pooping or pelvic pain.*

- PROLAPSE: *feeling like something is coming down or out of the vagina or anus*
- DIFFICULTY EMPTYING THE BOWEL: *this may also be related to poor coordination and spasming; learning to relax the pelvic floor may help*
- PELVIC PAIN: *pain in your bladder or bottom pre- and post-pooping, painful sex*

Bowel Massage

If you think about our intestine as being coated in muscle, it makes sense that massaging the intestine—in particular the large intestine, where things can get a little sluggish and gas can become trapped—can help soothe gut symptoms. This strategy is supported by a trial that demonstrated that daily bowel massage for eight weeks was an effective addition to managing both constipation and tummy pain.[62] The good thing about this type of massage is that it's free—you can easily do it yourself by following these simple steps, so why not give it a try? The bowel massage is best done daily, using massage oil.

> ✋ **Caution:** *If you are pregnant or have a history of inflammatory bowel disease, recent scarring, abdominal surgery, spine issues, or a history of colon cancer, it's best to discuss abdominal massage with your doctor first.*

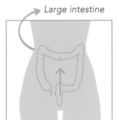
Large intestine

1. PREPARING THE GUT

Gently stroke upward with a flat hand (3 times).

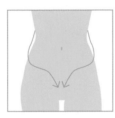

2. STIMULATING THE GUT

Stroke from your middle back firmly down the sides of your tummy into the groin (10 times).

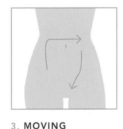

3. MOVING THINGS ALONG

Using your fists, stroke up and around your large intestine, with your right fist moving up and across, and your left fist moving down (2 minutes).

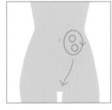

4. PUMPING DOWN

Using your fist, knead down the left side of your intestine. Imagine you're kneading dough down a tube (2 minutes).

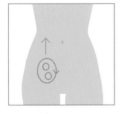

5. MOVING THINGS UP

Follow the instructions for step 4, but move up the right intestine instead (2 minutes).

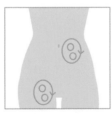

6. FINAL PUSH

Repeat step 4 and then step 3.

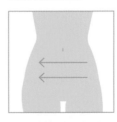

7. WINDING DOWN

Gently stroke across with a flat hand (10 times).

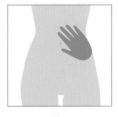

8. GAS RELEASE

Gently push down and shake with a flat hand across the large intestine (6 spots).

CHAPTER 8

Your Gut-Health
Action Plan

Your Gut-Health Journey Starts Here

This is where change begins and results are achieved. This section is all about personalizing this book to reflect your very own unique gut-health journey and goals; no two people will be the same. We'll bring together all the knowledge you've taken the time to learn from this book, and the assessments you have completed, to help prioritize and plan your next steps.

Consider this space your activity pad—this is where you can record the results from each of the assessments, along with any of the specific strategies that you feel are relevant and feasible for you. You can also jot down any extra notes to help consolidate different concepts from the book. There is no wrong or right way of doing this: You can complete as many or as few of the sections as you wish, and whether you start today or in a few months, again, it's completely your call. As with all of the assessments, you'll find a PDF of Your Gut-Health Action Plan template at theguthealthdoctor.com/book. You may find it useful to complete the assessments once at the beginning of your journey and again when some time has passed.

> ## Making Time
>
> *If you find yourself delaying things because you feel you just don't have the time, I want you to stop for a moment and imagine life with fewer sick days and more productive days, without those gut issues, or even just feeling that little bit happier and more focused. Think of the time you would save, time you could reinvest into your family, friends, hobbies, work, or just you. Even if you start by spending just a few minutes each day implementing one of your strategies, isn't it worth a try?*

Record your results from each assessment as you go through the book to help keep track of how things are progressing.

STEP 1:

Listening to Your Gut Feelings
(page 21)

Taking the time to pinpoint any specific gut symptoms that are bothering you is an important first step to bringing about change. The type, location, frequency, and severity of symptoms can help you select the right strategies to beat your symptoms for good.

DATE: ....

GUT-SYMPTOM SCORE:................................

KEY SYMPTOMS:..

DO YOU HAVE ANY ALARM FEATURES? ....

....

....

....

....

STRATEGIES: ....

....

....

....

....

....

REVIEW DATE: ....

STEP 2:

Checking In with Your Poop
(page 24)

OK, so it's not something we need to start discussing over dinner, but your poop is an invaluable resource when it comes to assessing your gut health. Inspecting every "delivery" is certainly not required; instead, just keep an eye on what your average poop looks like.

DATE: ....

FREQUENCY: ....

TIME OF DAY:...

CONSISTENCY: ....

COLOR: ....

AVERAGE DAILY POOP SIZE: ....

DO YOU HAVE ANY ALARM FEATURES?...................

....

STRATEGIES: ....

....

....

....

....

REVIEW DATE: ....

STEP 3:

How Diverse Is Your GM?

(page 35)

Our diet offers unique insight into our GM diversity. Because, after all, our microbes are completely reliant on what we feed them. Rest assured, we don't need to sacrifice taste and flavor, but just sparing a thought for our microbes at each meal can go a long way to improving not just their health and happiness but ours, too.

DATE: ....

FIBER SCORE: ....

DIET-DERIVED GM SCORE: ....

STRATEGIES (DON'T FORGET THOSE FROM YOUR PLANT-BASED DIVERSITY PLANNER ON PAGE 81):

....

....

....

....

....

....

....

REVIEW DATE: ....

STEP 4:

How Happy Are You?

(page 41)

There is no escaping the link between our gut and our brain. And now, with trials demonstrating the impact of a "gut-boosting" diet on mental health, there's a strong case for checking in with your happiness levels before and after implementing the strategies within this book.

DATE: ....

SCORE: ....

STRATEGIES: ....

....

....

REVIEW DATE: ....

STEP 5:

Gut-Brain Assessment

(page 89)

For those who experience a collection of gut symptoms, it can be helpful to assess whether the gut-brain axis is involved in perpetuating them. Determining this will inform the most effective pathway needed to manage your symptoms.

DATE: ....

SCORE: ....

STRATEGIES: ....

....

....

REVIEW DATE: ....

STEP 6:

Are Food Intolerances to Blame?
(page 126)

Determining whether a food is the cause of your symptoms can be incredibly confusing. Instead, taking a systematic, evidence-based approach using the 3R Method can help cut through the misperceptions and fear attached to certain foods. This process will help to reestablish your relationship with food by getting to the bottom of suspected food intolerances, in turn empowering you to enjoy more foods with confidence.

DATE: ....

RESULT OF STEP 1: RECORD: ....

....

RESULT OF STEP 2: RESTRICT: ....

....

RESULT OF STEP 3: REINTRODUCE:.....................

....

....

....

PLAN: ....

....

....

REVIEW DATE: ....

STEP 7:

Is It IBS or Another Functional Gut Disorder?
(page 145)

I'm not generally one for labels, but getting the right diagnosis is key to getting your symptoms under control. This is because it eliminates a lot of the trial and error, allowing you to choose more targeted strategies based on trials in people with the same diagnosis.

DATE: ....

DO YOU NEED TO SEE YOUR DOCTOR?
If so, record date of appointment:

....

HAVE YOU BEEN TESTED FOR CELIAC DISEASE AND OTHER OVERLAPPED DISEASES?
Record date and test results:

....

DO YOU FULFILL IBS CRITERIA? ....

IBS SUBTYPE: ....

DO YOU HAVE ANOTHER FUNCTIONAL GUT DISORDER?

....

STRATEGIES: ....

....

....

....

RESULT OF STAGE 1: RESTRICTION..

....

RESULT OF STAGE 2: REINTRODUCTION..

....

RESULT OF STAGE 3: PERSONALIZATION..

....

STEP 8:
Let's Talk About Sleep
(page 172)

Although it may sound like a no-brainer, too few of us are getting enough good-quality sleep. As we explored, improving your sleep can have far-reaching benefits, extending to diet, immunity, mood, and focus. With that in mind, it's certainly worth considering your sleeping habits and testing out some of the sleep-hygiene strategies.

DATE: ....

SCORE: ....

STRATEGIES: ....

....

....

....

....

REVIEW DATE: ....

STEP 9:
How Good Is Your Immunity?
(page 174)

Are you constantly getting sick? It could be a tell-tale sign that you need to check in with your GM—how are you treating it? Yes, when it comes to your immunity, there are factors outside your control. But there are also a number of factors within your control: Diet, sleep, stress, and exercise all play an important part.

DATE: ....

SCORE: ....

STRATEGIES: ....

....

....

....

....

REVIEW DATE: ....

STEP 10:

Is Stress Getting the Best of You?

(page 178)

We've all experienced stress, and that's normal. But when it becomes a regular occurrence, it can seriously affect your health and happiness. No one should have to live with the consequences of stress overload but, unfortunately, many of us do. Is stress affecting you?

DATE: ....

SCORE: ....

STRATEGIES: ....

....

....

....

....

....

REVIEW DATE: ....

STEP 11:

How Active Are You?

(page 191)

You may always be rushing around and feel physically exhausted, but have you ever stopped and considered how your fitness levels stack up against recommendations? Sometimes it just takes a quick check for us to realize that we've got caught up in the daily grind, sporting a racing mind and an inactive body.

DATE: ....

SCORE: ....

STRATEGIES: ....

....

....

REVIEW DATE: ....

WHAT ABOUT YOUR BOWEL FITNESS AND TECHNIQUE?

(pages 194 to 196)

....

ARE YOU A GOOD POOPER? ....

HOW STRONG IS YOUR PELVIC FLOOR?

....

....

STRATEGIES: ....

....

....

REVIEW DATE: ....

Forming New Habits

Forming healthy habits isn't always easy. We often start with the best intentions but, within a few weeks or so, when the motivation starts to fade and the demands of life take over, we can find ourselves back at square one. To help combat this common pattern that can affect us all, I've listed my top habit-forming tips, which have been tried and tested by my patients.

- Form a trigger by attaching the activity to another habit, e.g., brushing your teeth.

- Set a daily reminder on your phone until the action becomes automatic.

- If you're into lists, start a daily checklist.

- Keep the time and place consistent.

- Find a friend who may also benefit; you can then keep each other motivated.

- Leave a sticky note on your bedroom mirror reminding you why you started.

- Record any good feelings or experiences related to the activity in a notepad.

- Celebrating any success, no matter how small, can really help reinforce your commitment.

- Don't be too hard on yourself if you miss a day or two; look forward to getting back to it tomorrow.

- Be realistic from the start: Don't try to implement too many changes at once. If the activity calls for fifteen minutes a day but you only have ten minutes, just start with that. If it means you get started today, you'll still be one step ahead.

- If your motivation is running on empty, try bringing some emotion back into the activity by asking yourself two questions:

1

How will I feel if I continue versus if I stop?

2

What will my life look like in one year if I continue versus if I stop?

Set Your Goals

So there you have it—the foundation of your gut-health journey has been laid. It's really only the start but, undoubtedly, that's a victory in itself and something you should be unashamedly proud of. You've made a conscious decision to take charge of your health and happiness by beginning this journey of self-discovery and getting to know your GM and all its mind-blowing potential. With the intention of condensing and prioritizing all the things you've learned along the way, think about what your top three gut-health goals for the next six months might be.

Goal 1: Notes:	
Goal 2: Notes:	
Goal 3: Notes:	

Over time, these may change, but setting targets for yourself can keep you focused on what's most important to you.

CHAPTER 9

In the Kitchen

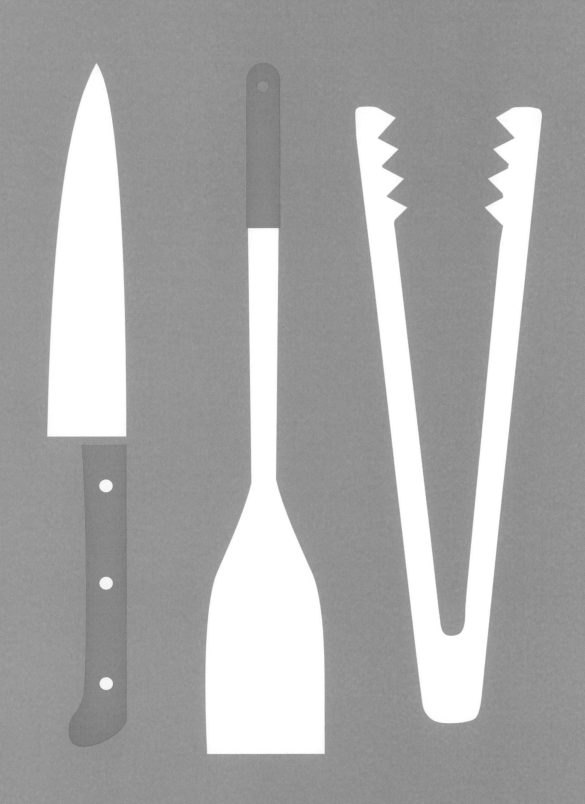

In the Kitchen

Welcome to my kitchen, my favorite room in the house. This is where I see small changes make a big impact. My kitchen mission is to translate the science from lab to plate, creating delicious food that won't just make your taste buds dance but will see your gut microbes thrive, too.

Food makes me very happy—I come from a big Italian family, where mealtimes are celebrations that bring all my favorite people together. But I know it's not the same for everyone. For many of my patients, who lead busy lives or are struggling with gut issues, the thought of preparing food can provoke added stress and anxiety. If this sounds like you, I want this chapter to help change that for you. This is about reviving your passion for flavor and food; I want you to feel at ease with these recipes. They offer flexibility with intolerances, time limitations, space constraints, budgets, cooking skills—inclusivity is the name of my cooking game. I've also included my beginner's guide to fermenting and sprouting—two of my favorite activities, which really do open up a whole other world of food, flavor, and fun.

To start, let's revisit the concept of "gut-friendly" food. This is a rather ambiguous term because it can mean different things to different people. For example, for those without gut symptoms whose primary goal is to boost beneficial microbes, many high-FODMAP foods (which, as we discussed in chapter 6, are high in prebiotics) are great to include. But for those with irritable bowel syndrome (IBS), large amounts may trigger symptoms. To help with this, I've added tips on how to modify the recipes, making it easy to turn any of them into a dish that fits your dietary needs. Keep in mind that many of the restrictions we discussed in chapters 4, 5, and 6 are only short-term tools to help identify your triggers or to give your gut a little rest while you work on settling that gut-brain axis using the strategies we looked at in chapter 7.

The underlying theme of all the recipes is that they provide good nutrition for both you and your gut microbiota (GM), so whether the recipe is low in lactose or gluten-free, rest assured, neither your taste buds nor your GM will be missing out.

Meal Planning: Building the Foundation

Although it's not for everyone, meal planning can be a valuable tool in terms of overcoming barriers to nourishing you and your microbes. If you're struggling with this, you'll recognize that no amount of knowledge can overcome it; planning really is key. I'm certainly not talking about generic meal plans—in my ten years of experience, I've yet to meet anyone who has succeeded with one. Yes, perhaps you can stick to it for a few weeks but, as soon as life gets busy, it's usually the first thing to go. My no-generic-meal-plan approach is not always popular when I first suggest it to patients who walk in with their heart set on one. However, they quickly discover that a generic plan simply doesn't work, and it's because only you know the ins and outs of your life. You're the only one who can create a plan that works for you.

But don't worry, you're not on your own: This chapter offers guidance and inspiration to help get you started. On the next page is the template that my patients who are struggling with this barrier use to create their own tailored plans. You'll see that I've also included a space to record your planning and shopping. I know this may sound a little regimented but, for many, having this structure for around nine weeks (remember: it's thought that's the average time to form a habit, according to research from University College London) can turn meal planning from feeling like a taxing obligation into second nature. Looking after your GM is a marathon, not a sprint—we're looking for long-term changes. However, if you prefer to start off with a sprint, to build your motivation and momentum, by all means sprint away—just keep a gauge on your fuel tank along the way.

I have filled out Monday as an example of what one day might look like.

	Breakfast	Lunch	Dinner	Snacks*	Drinks
Monday	*DIY Granola (page 225)*	*Mix-and-Match Sliders (page 234)*	*Meatless Meatballs in Rich Tomato Sauce (page 258)*	*Sea Salt and Rosemary Legume Crunch (page 270)*	*Water (50 ounces/1.5 L)* *1 shot of coffee* *Water Kefir (page 302)*
Tuesday					
Wednesday					
Thursday					
Friday					
Saturday					
Sunday					
Plant points**					
Planning day			**Shopping day**		

Remember to be realistic: Include some of your faves.

***Did you reach your thirty different plant-based foods? Remember, from chapter 3, that our GM craves plant diversity.*

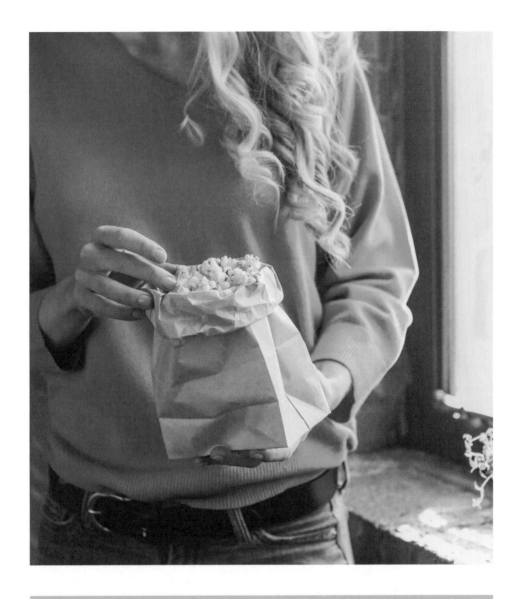

Snacks on the run

- *Naked fruit*
- *Naked nuts and seeds*
- *Live natural yogurt*
- *Popcorn au naturel*

As a general guide, products with at least 3 g fiber/100 g, no added sugar in the ingredients list, and salt content of 0.3 g/100 g or less (or sodium 0.1 g/100 g or less).

Recipe Modifications

Modification	Ingredient	Replacement
GLUTEN-FREE	Soy sauce	• Tamari (double-check on the label that it doesn't contain wheat) • Gluten-free soy sauce
	Baking powder	• Gluten-free baking powder
	Grains/pasta	• Gluten-free grains, such as amaranth, buckwheat, legumes, millet, oats, quinoa, whole-grain rice
	Spelt, whole wheat flour	• Whole-grain gluten-free flour • Combine 50 percent brown rice flour, 25 percent cornstarch, 25 percent almond meal
FODMAP-lite* * See page 160 for the FODMAP-lite approach. For those following the full FODMAP approach, see your dietitian for a comprehensive list of high- and low-FODMAP foods.	Garlic, onion	• Pickled • Garlic-infused oil (store-bought) • Asafetida powder (best "fried off" in the pan with a touch of oil before adding other ingredients) • Green part of scallion • Chives
	Additional herbs and spices	• Allspice, basil, capers, cinnamon, coriander, cumin, curry powder, dill, ginger, lemon, lime, mint, mustard, nutmeg, paprika, parsley, pepper, rosemary, thyme, turmeric, and vanilla
LOW-LACTOSE		See page 135
DAIRY-FREE	Yogurt	Plant-based yogurt (coconut, soy, etc.)
	Cow's milk	Plant-based milks** (soy, rice, oat, almond) ***Opt for calcium-fortified. Cow's milk cannot be substituted with plant-based milks in the fermenting recipes.*

Modification	Ingredient	Replacement
OTHER	Self-rising flour	1 cup/120 g plain flour + 1 teaspoon baking powder
	Egg	• (for binding) **Flax egg:** 1 tablespoon ground flaxseed with 3 tablespoons warm water; stir and let set for 15 minutes • (for binding) **Chia egg:** 1 tablespoon chia seeds with 3 tablespoons warm water; stir and let set for 15 minutes • (for thickening) **Arrowroot:** 1 tablespoon • (most purposes) **Egg replacer** (made from blended flours, raising agents, and gums): available from most health-food shops
	Nuts	• **Toppings:** Legume Crunch (page 270), crumbled seeded crackers (page 269), dried fruit • **Butters:** sunflower seed, pumpkin seed • **Coatings:** cornmeal, rolled oats, bread crumbs • **Added texture:** finely diced celery, bean sprouts, chopped scallion
	Cheese	• Cashew Cheese (page 237) • Other plant-based cheeses (soy, almond, etc.) • Nutritional yeast***

***What's the deal with nutritional yeast? Although it's similar to the yeast used to make bread and brew beer, the function of nutritional yeast is very different. The yeast is not alive, so it doesn't do any fermenting. Instead, it is used to add flavor (a delicious cheesy, nutty taste) and nutrition. Nutritional yeast is an excellent source of B vitamins (including B_{12}, when fortified) and is rich in fiber and protein. Because of this, fortified nutritional yeast is considered a dietary staple for those whose diet is 100 percent plant-based.

PART 2

Recipes

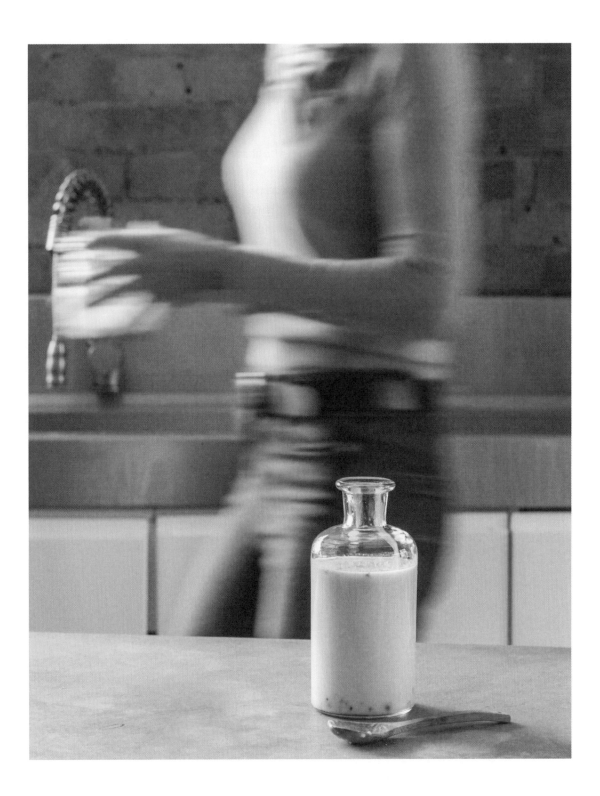

Breakfast

For me, there really is something special about breakfast. Whether it's creamy kefir oats, some granola crunch, light and fluffy pancakes, perfectly gooey eggs, or a warm breakfast loaf, it's all part of my breakfast love affair. For those who need a bit more convincing, breakfast not only physically sets your gut up for the day, triggering that gastrocolic reflex (which gets "things" moving), if you're feeding your GM (think fiber, plant diversity), breakfast has been shown to increase mental and physical alertness, too. Psychologically, kicking your day off with a nutritious start can lay down a strong, positive foundation for the rest of the day. For those who are still a little unsure, keep in mind that there are no breakfast rules—it doesn't need to be big if you're not hungry or eaten as soon as you wake up if you're into the longer fasts. You can also prevent it from becoming a time-consuming, full-on event if your mornings are a little chaotic, with my Breakfast on the Run options. Do breakfast your way, just try not to miss out on what it has to offer.

Fermented Overnight Oats (My Breakfast Staple)

There's something comforting about going to bed knowing that millions of microbes will continue working through the night, transforming your breakfast into a flavor-infused jar of goodness. As the microbes from the kefir prepare your breakfast, that is, ferment it, they produce beneficial organic acids, which are a little tart-tasting. I crave that tart bite, but if you're new to fermenting you may want to shorten the fermenting time and build up. This recipe works best with homemade kefir from grains (see Dairy Kefir; page 300), but you can use store-bought as well. And this recipe doesn't just offer live microbes; it also provides a sizeable 8 grams of fiber per portion.

Overnight Oats

½ cup (45 g) rolled oats
1 teaspoon mixed seeds, such as flaxseed, sunflower, pumpkin, and sesame
1 tablespoon chia seeds
1 tablespoon unsweetened shredded coconut
1 extra-ripe banana, peeled and mashed (3.5 ounces/100 g)
¼ cup (60 ml) Dairy Kefir (page 300; see Note)
¾ cup plus 1 tablespoon (200 ml) soy milk, or milk of choice
1 Medjool date, thinly chopped, or sweetener of choice

Toppings (choose 1)

CARROT CAKE
½ small carrot, grated (1.5 ounces/40 g)
1 tablespoon walnuts, crushed
½ teaspoon cinnamon

COCOA AND ZUCCHINI
¼ small zucchini, grated (1.5 ounces/40 g)
2 teaspoons cocoa powder
1 tablespoon dark chocolate shavings

1. In a mixing bowl, combine all the ingredients for the overnight oats and toppings of choice and stir well.

2. Divide into two 12-ounce (or 300 ml) jars and cover with lids.

3. Leave in a warm (around 80°F/25°C), dark place overnight to allow the kefir microbes to work their magic, infusing the flavors throughout.

4. After 8 hours, stir through. Breakfast is served! Pop the second jar in the fridge for tomorrow's breakfast.

Not ready for fermenting? Replace the kefir with your milk of choice and leave in the fridge overnight.

Breakfast on the Run

Serves 1

Don't let those manic mornings get in the way of a tasty and nutritious breakfast for you and your GM. These are some of my fast favorites that have saved me from many sugar-overloaded breakfast bars and store-bought buttery pastries that never quite seem to hit the mark.

MONDAY

Two-Minute Scramble

1 teaspoon olive oil
2 large eggs, whisked
2 tablespoons milk
1 tablespoon fresh herbs or scallions, finely chopped
1 slice grainy bread, roughly chopped
6 cherry tomatoes, halved
Salt
Fresh ground black pepper
Mixed seeds, such as flaxseed, sunflower, pumpkin, and sesame (optional)

1. Swirl one large mug (or bowl) with the oil, then add the eggs, milk, herbs, bread, and tomatoes. Season with salt and pepper and shake in the mixed seeds, if using. Roughly mix. The egg will rise when cooking so ensure the mug/bowl is no more than half full.

2. Cook on high in the microwave for 1 minute. Stir. Return to the microwave for 1 more minute or until the egg has set.

TUESDAY

Live Breakfast Parfait

¾ cup (200 g) Probiotic Yogurt (page 306)
½ cup (50 g) berries of choice
⅓ cup (40 g) DIY Granola (page 225)
1 tablespoon dark chocolate, shaved

1. Spoon half the yogurt into a tall serving glass, then add half the berries, then half the granola, and repeat.

2. Top with chocolate shavings.

WEDNESDAY

Thick Protein Shake

4 ounces (110 g) silken tofu
1 large banana, frozen
1 cup (240 ml) Dairy Kefir (page 300)
1 teaspoon ground cinnamon
Mixed seeds, such as flaxseed, sunflower, pumpkin, and sesame (optional)
1 tablespoon DIY Granola (page 225, optional)

Put the tofu, banana, kefir, and cinammon in a blender and buzz until smooth. (If it's too thick, add some milk of choice; alternatively, just eat it like ice cream!) Top with the mixed seeds and granola, if using.

THURSDAY

Avocado and Feta Slider

½ medium tomato, thinly sliced
¼ avocado, thinly sliced
2 whole-grain crackers (see options on page 269)
¼ cup (30 g) crumbled feta
Mixed seeds, such as flaxseed, sunflower, pumpkin, and sesame
Salt
Fresh ground black pepper

Lay the tomato slices on top of the crackers, then layer on the avocado. Sprinkle with the feta and seeds, and season to taste with salt and pepper.

Peanut and Pear Open Sandwich

2 tablespoons peanut
   butter
1 pear, cut lengthwise
   into 6 or 7 slices
2 tablespoons Probiotic
   Yogurt (page 306)
Mixed seeds, such as
   flaxseed, sunflower,
   pumpkin, and sesame

Spread the peanut
butter across a slice of
pear, add some yogurt,
and top with seeds. Eat
and repeat.

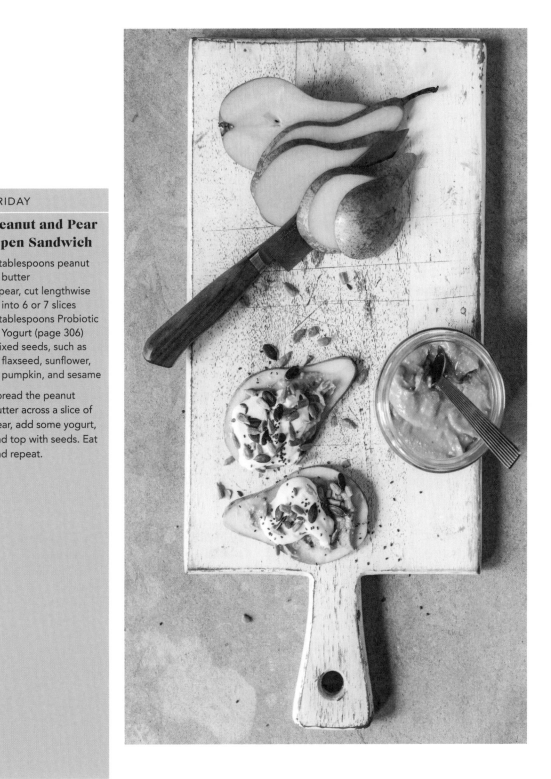

Mix-and-Match Porridge

Many of us tend to eat the same breakfast on repeat, making it a rather boring meal. This DIY breakfast template is all about inspiring you to mix things up and get creative. Build the ultimate breakfast by choosing one ingredient per box. Stir together and enjoy! The portions are just there as a guide, but remember it's your breakfast!

Fiber Base   (1.5 ounces/40 g)
The base way to kick things off

Raw grains typically double in size when cooked; if starting with raw, use 1.5 ounces (40 g). If choosing cooked options, for ultimate convenience, use precooked grains (3 ounces/80 g), which require no more than 1 to 2 minutes in the microwave; otherwise, cook according to the package instructions.

- Rolled oats (scant ½ cup raw)
- Rolled wheat flakes (⅓ cup raw)
- Buckwheat hot cereal (¼ cup raw)
- Amaranth (¼ cup raw)
- Quinoa (¼ cup raw)

Flavor Punch
Reward your taste buds for getting you out of bed

- Coconut flakes (1 tablespoon) & vanilla extract (¼ teaspoon)
- Ground cinnamon (½ teaspoon) & nutmeg (pinch)
- Grated ginger & ground cinnamon (½ teaspoon each)
- Dark chocolate chips (1 tablespoon)
- Crumbled feta cheese (1 tablespoon)

Live Culture   (2 tablespoons)
Add some microbes to your mix

- Probiotic Yogurt (page 306)
- Dairy Kefir (page 300)
- Plain probiotic coconut yogurt
- Coconut kefir
- Kimchi (page 296)

Polyphenol Hit
(⅓ cup/50 g)
GM-loving plant chemicals

- Sliced strawberries
- Blueberries
- Grated apple
- Sliced pear
- Chickpeas
- Cherry tomatoes

Hydration
(½ to ⅓ cups/120 to 160 ml)
After all, our body is over 50 percent water

- Cow's milk
- Soy milk*
- Oat milk*
- Almond milk*
- Side of tea

Consider opting for calcium-fortified varieties.

Prebiotic Boost
(1 tablespoon)
A real treat for the best-behaved microbes

- Dried figs, thinly sliced
- Dates or prunes, thinly sliced
- Dried apricots, diced
- Cashews
- Pomegranate

Healthy Fats
(1 tablespoon)
Fuel a healthy heart and mind

- Walnuts
- Almond butter
- Pistachios
- Chia seeds
- Avocado

Plant Power Pancakes

Breakfast is often a missed opportunity when it comes to contributing to your five portions of vegetables per day—and these pancakes will put a stop to that. But they don't just deliver on veggies; they're also a real treat for the taste buds.

Pancakes

1 medium sweet potato (about 5 ounces/150 g), roughly chopped

⅔ cup (60 g) rolled oats

⅓ cup (75 g) drained and rinsed canned cannellini beans

1 large extra-ripe banana, peeled (4 ounces/120 g)

1 cup (240 ml) soy milk, or milk of choice

4 large eggs, whisked

1 teaspoon ground cinnamon

1 teaspoon vanilla extract

1 teaspoon baking powder

Olive oil, or oil of choice, for frying

Berry Sauce

1 cup (160 g) diced strawberries

1 Medjool date, chopped

To serve

½ cup (120 g) Probiotic Yogurt (page 306)

1 tablespoon mixed seeds, such as flaxseed, sunflower, pumpkin, and sesame

1. To prepare the pancakes, place the sweet potato and a small splash of water in a microwave-safe dish. Cover and cook on high for 4 minutes. Remove and let cool.

2. To prepare the berry sauce, combine the strawberries, date, and ½ cup (120 ml) water in a small saucepan and bring to a gentle boil. Using the back of a spatula, squish the strawberries and date, then simmer for 10 minutes.

3. Meanwhile, once the sweet potato has cooled, blend together with all the remaining pancake ingredients, except the oil, to form a smooth batter.

4. In a nonstick frying pan, warm a little oil over medium-low heat. Pour in ¼ cup (60 ml) of the batter and cook for 3 minutes or so, until there are bubbles in the pancake and you can lift it to flip easily.

5. Flip and cook on the other side for 1 to 2 minutes. Transfer to a plate and cover with a clean cloth to keep warm.

6. Repeat the process with the rest of the batter. Serve the pancakes drizzled with the berry sauce, yogurt, and mixed seeds.

Oats are a great source of beta-glucans, a type of fiber. There is strong evidence for their health benefits, which include lowering cholesterol and managing sugar levels in people with diabetes. They've also been shown to help regulate our appetite, making us less likely to grab for the cookie jar.

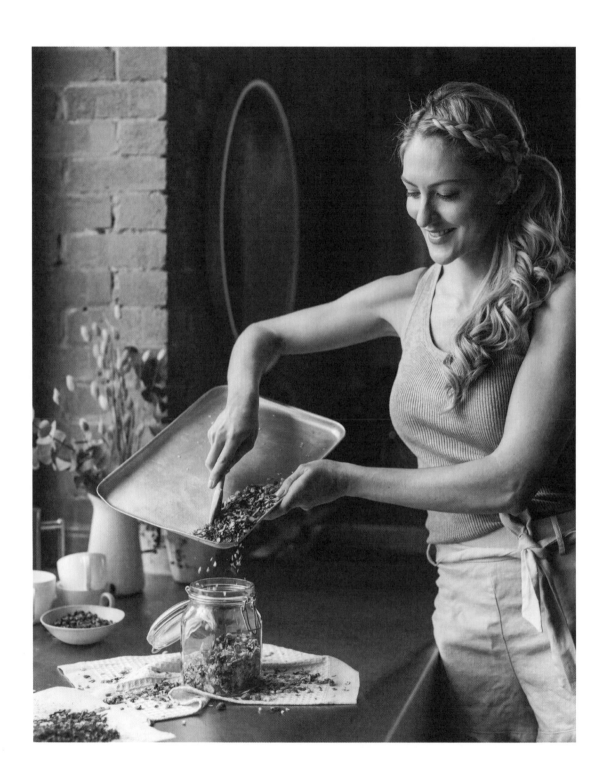

DIY Granola

After searching high and low, I still couldn't find a granola that checked the boxes for both flavor and nutrition. So I decided to make my own gut-loving mix, and I haven't looked back! I make a batch every other Sunday and use it as both a breakfast and a snack, adding that all-important crunch to my yogurt. Each portion also provides close to a third of your daily fiber needs. Serve this granola with Probiotic Yogurt (page 183) or milk of your choice.

Granola

Generous 1 cup (110 g) rolled oats (or muesli mix of choice)
½ cup (70 g) almonds, chopped
½ cup (70 g) mixed seeds, such as flaxseed, sunflower, pumpkin, and sesame
⅓ cup (20 g) coconut flakes
1½ teaspoons olive oil
½ teaspoon ground cinnamon
½ teaspoon ground nutmeg
½ teaspoon vanilla extract
2 Medjool dates, stirred into a paste with 1 tablespoon boiling water, or sweetener of choice
2 teaspoons ground ginger (optional)

Toppings (optional)

One 15-ounce (425 g) can lentils, drained and rinsed
1 medium raw beet, grated
¼ cup (25 g) dried goji berries
5 dried figs (about 45 g), sliced
8 dried apricots (about 55 g), sliced

1. Preheat the oven to 325°F (165°C). Line two baking sheets with parchment paper.

2. In a large bowl, combine the oats, almonds, seeds, and coconut.

3. In a small bowl, mix together the oil, cinnamon, nutmeg, vanilla, and dates, and the ginger, if using, before pouring over the dry ingredients. Using your hands, mix together to coat evenly. Set aside.

4. Thinly spread the mix across the prepared baking sheets. Pop in the oven for 10 minutes, toss, then continue baking for another 10 minutes, or until golden. If you are including the lentils or beet, pat dry before laying on separate baking sheets, and place in the oven alongside the granola mix (20 minutes for the beet, 30 minutes for the lentils, or until dry and crisp).

5. Remove the granola from the oven and sprinkle on your toppings of choice. Allow to cool before placing in an airtight container, where it will keep for two weeks.

VARIATIONS

• Like a chunkier granola? Add 2 tablespoons water and double the oil and dates. Press into the tray and bake for an extra 5 to 10 minutes.

• Experiment with different grains, nuts, and dried fruits to introduce more diversity into your diet.

The phytochemical betalain that is found in beets is what you have to thank for turning your cereal milk pink. Better still, betalain has been shown to be a powerful antioxidant with anticancer properties, at least in animal studies.

Chickpea Crêpes with Creamy Feta and Fungi

Proof that a glamorous dish full of flavor doesn't need to cost you your whole morning in prep or cleaning—it really is the perfect way to start your weekend. While the batter rests, consider doing your morning yoga flow (see page 183).

Crêpes
⅓ cup plus 2 tablespoons (50 g) chickpea flour (gram or besan flour)
½ teaspoon garlic powder
Pinch of salt
Fresh ground black pepper
0.5 ounce (15 g) pickled beet greens or spinach leaves
Olive oil, or oil of choice, for frying

Toppings
1 tablespoon olive oil
7 ounces (200 g) mushrooms, chopped
1 garlic clove, thinly sliced
¼ teaspoon fresh rosemary or thyme leaves (optional)
¼ cup (60 g) Probiotic Yogurt (page 306) or Classic Hummus (page 264)
¼ cup (40 g) crumbled feta
1 cup (150 g) cherry tomatoes, halved
Sprinkle of seeds
Poached egg or slice of smoked salmon (optional)

1. To make the crêpe batter, place the flour, garlic powder, salt, pepper, pickled greens, and ½ cup (120 ml) water to a blender. Blend for 30 seconds. Set the thin batter aside for 30 minutes in a warm place to allow the flour to hydrate while you prep the toppings.

2. To prepare the toppings, heat the oil in a frying pan over medium heat, then add the mushrooms and garlic. Stir together and sauté for 2 to 3 minutes, until soft and slightly browned. Add any optional fresh herbs and season to taste.

3. To cook the crêpes, warm a little oil in a nonstick frying pan over medium heat. Add ⅓ cup (80 ml) of the batter to the pan.

4. Cook for 2 to 3 minutes, until there are bubbles in the crêpe and you can lift it over to flip easily.

5. Flip and cook on the other side for 1 to 2 minutes.

6. Transfer to a plate and cover with a clean cloth to keep warm. Repeat the process with the remaining batter.

7. Line your crêpe with a dollop of yogurt or hummus, a layer of warm mushrooms, and a crumble of feta. Top with some tomatoes, seeds, and egg or salmon, if desired, before folding the crêpe and digging in.

Similarly to the way in which our skin can make vitamin D when exposed to sunlight, so, too, can mushrooms. In the winter, I keep my mushrooms on my kitchen window sill, exposed to sunlight, to maximize my vitamin D intake. Vitamin D is crucial not only for strong bones but for our mental health, too.

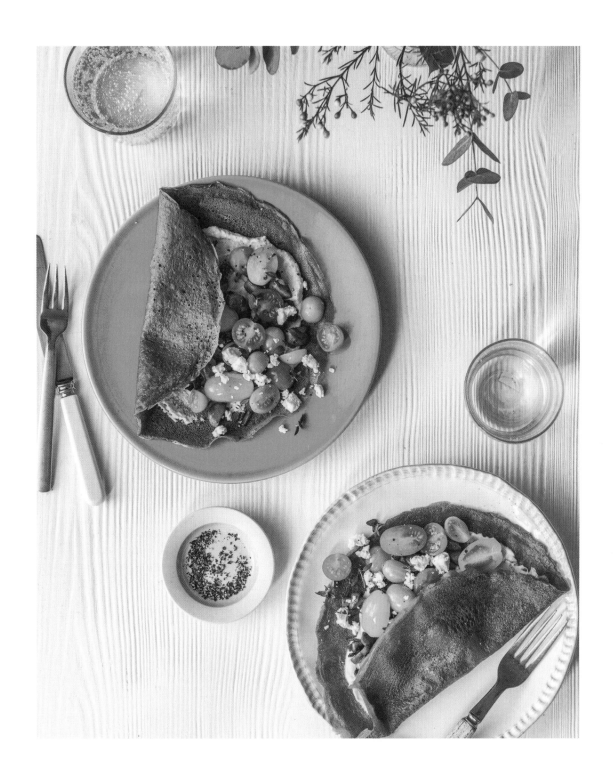

Mini Shakshuka Egg Pots

After making these beauties, you'll never be tempted to order baked eggs out again.

3 bell peppers, mixed colors
1 tablespoon olive oil
6 scallions, chopped
4 garlic cloves, thinly sliced
1 teaspoon cumin seeds
¾ cup (200 g) drained and rinsed canned butter beans
6 medium tomatoes, chopped
1 handful cilantro, chopped
2 tablespoons black olives, chopped (optional)
2 tablespoons capers (optional)
Red pepper flakes
Salt
Fresh ground black pepper
4 small whole wheat tortillas
4 large eggs
3 tablespoons Probiotic Yogurt (page 306)
Seeded crackers (optional; see pages 267 to 269)

1. Preheat the oven to 375°F (190°C).

2. Grill the peppers in a griddle pan over high heat for approximately 15 minutes, turning frequently until nice and charred on both sides. Set aside and, when cooled, chop into small pieces.

3. Warm the oil in a nonstick frying pan over medium heat. Add the scallions, garlic, and cumin. Fry until soft and slightly browned. Add the beans, tomatoes, grilled peppers, cilantro, and the olives and capers, if using, and season to taste with red pepper flakes, salt, and black pepper. Simmer for 10 to 15 minutes, until soft. You may need to add a little water if the mixture gets too dry.

4. Line each of four 8-ounce (240 ml) ramekins (or ovenproof mugs) with a tortilla.

5. Divide the shakshuka between each ramekin, make a well in the middle, and crack an egg into each one.

6. Place the ramekins on a baking sheet and bake for 8 to 10 minutes, until the whites are set but the yolks are still runny. Top with a dollop of yogurt and enjoy warm with crackers to dip in, if desired.

Ever wondered why some egg yolks are darker than others? The delicious deep-orange color is all thanks to the higher levels of the phytochemical beta-carotene. Studies have found that free-range chickens often produce eggs with higher levels of beta-carotene, as well as other nutrients, such as omega-3. Why? Free-range chickens graze not only on grass, seeds, and weeds but also on worms and insects, which makes their diet more nutrient dense.

Spicy Baked Beans

I didn't think I was that into baked beans until my friend Niki (who I call the flavor queen) opened my eyes. Now I always make a double batch and add them into my Mix-and-Match Gut-Goodness Bowls (page 246) the next day. I also freeze them into single portions and reheat as a snack. In terms of prebiotic load, this dish is hard to beat, and it sports 10 grams of total fiber per portion.

Baked Beans
2 tablespoons olive oil
1 onion, diced
3 garlic cloves, crushed
1 teaspoon cumin seeds
1 teaspoon smoked
    paprika
½ teaspoon cayenne pepper
One 14.5-ounce (411 g) can
    whole peeled tomatoes
4 sun-dried tomatoes,
    preserved in oil
One 15-ounce (425 g) can
    cranberry or Roman
    beans, drained and rinsed
One 15-ounce (425 g) can
    cannellini beans, drained
    and rinsed
¼ cup (40 g) pitted black
    olives, sliced (optional)
1 tablespoon tamari or soy
    sauce
1 teaspoon sweetener of
    choice
1 teaspoon vinegar of choice
1⅓ cups/40 g spinach
    (optional)
1 teaspoon red pepper
    flakes (optional)
Salt
Fresh ground black pepper

Toppings (optional)
8 eggs, poached, fried, or
    scrambled
Probiotic Yogurt (page 306)
    or Classic Hummus (page
    264)
Small handful alfalfa
    sprouts (see page 304)

1. Warm the oil in a nonstick frying pan over medium-low heat. Add the onion, garlic, and spices and sauté for a few minutes.

2. Add the canned tomatoes and sun-dried tomatoes and simmer for 15 minutes over low heat.

3. Add the beans, and olives, if using, and cook for an additional 15 minutes.

4. Finally, add the tamari, sweetener, vinegar, and the spinach and red pepper flakes, if using. Simmer for a few minutes. Season to taste.

5. Plate the beans and, if desired, top with the eggs and a dollop of yogurt, hummus, or both. Sprinkle on the alfalfa sprouts, if using.

Considering skipping the oil? A trial compared the impact of eating cooked tomatoes with and without olive oil for five days. Those who included the oil had significantly greater levels of the phytochemical lycopene in their blood. Tomatoes + heat + olive oil = higher lycopene bioavailability. Why do we care about lycopene? Not only has it been shown to increase your skin's defense against the sun (although that's still not an excuse to skip sunscreen), it's also linked with better heart health and a lower risk of prostate cancer.

Serves 8

Banana, Fig, and Zucchini Breakfast Loaf

This is one of my favorite "accidental" creations. Throwing in a bit of this and a bit of that turned into something pretty magical. The loaf was devoured within an hour (I promise, I did share) and, thanks to all of your requests on social media, I decided to repeat the "accident" the next day, this time measuring out all the ingredients so that I could share it with you. Offering over 5 grams of fiber per portion, you'll be hard-pressed to find a loaf to match.

Loaf
1 cup (120 g) whole-grain spelt flour
½ cup (100 g) teff grains (see Note)
2 teaspoons baking powder
2 teaspoons ground cinnamon
Pinch of salt
3 large eggs
2½ tablespoons olive oil
2 teaspoons vanilla extract
3 extra-ripe bananas, peeled and mashed (1⅓ cups/300 g)
10 dried figs (about 70 g), diced
1 large carrot, grated (1 cup/100 g)
½ small zucchini, grated (⅔ cup/80 g)
½ cup (50 g) walnuts, roughly chopped

Toppings
1 banana, peeled and halved lengthwise (100 g)
2 tablespoons coconut flakes (optional)

1. Preheat the oven to 375°F (190°C). Line a 9 x 5 inch (23 x 13 cm) loaf pan with parchment paper.

2. In a large mixing bowl, combine the spelt, teff, baking powder, cinnamon, and salt.

3. In a separate bowl, whisk together the eggs, oil, and vanilla with an electric mixer. Add the bananas, figs, carrot, zucchini, and walnuts. Fold in the dry mixture.

4. Pour the cake batter into the prepared pan. Top with the banana halves any way you like and sprinkle on the coconut, if using.

5. Pop in the oven for 70 minutes, or until cooked through. Cover with foil after 30 minutes of cooking to prevent burning the coconut. Allow to cool for 5 minutes in the pan, then lift it out with the parchment paper onto a wire rack to cool completely before cutting.

NOTE: *The teff grains add brilliant texture to the loaf, but if you can't find any, replace with ¾ cup plus 1 tablespoon (100 g) spelt flour.*

Teff is a traditional staple in Ethiopia. This tiny gluten-free grain packs quite a nutritional punch, offering 10 grams of protein and 7 grams of fiber per cooked cup. It has a slightly sweet taste, with undertones of cocoa and hazelnut. You can buy the grains and flour (I prefer the texture of the grains) from most health-food stores or readily online.

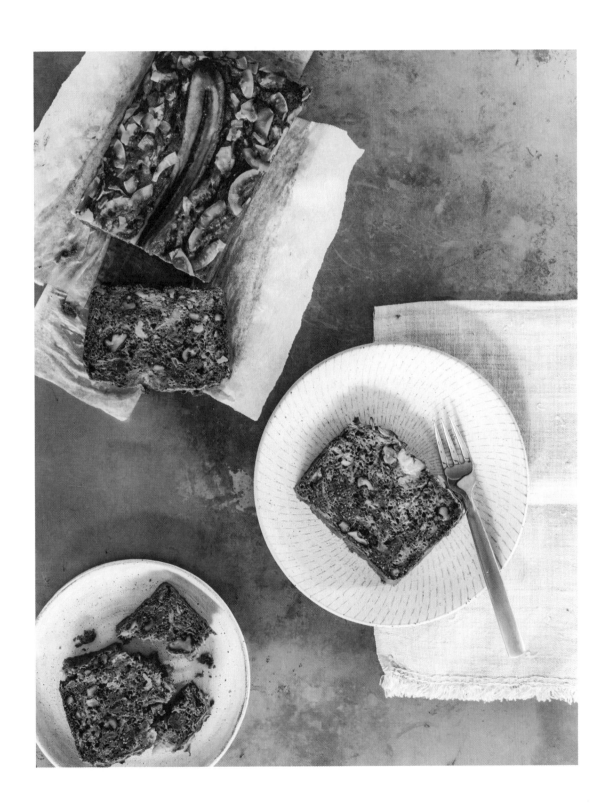

Lunch

Even if you don't live in a siesta-loving part of the world, lunch doesn't need to be a boring sandwich, a tasteless bag of leaves, or an expensive impulse buy. Here I share five-minute Mix-and-Match Slider ideas, convenient double-batch lunch-box recipes, and my GM-loving version of sushi that'll have you (and your colleagues) wishing you'd packed extras. For those times when you're looking for a more leisurely lunch that will have your guests raving for weeks, you may be tempted by the Korean BBQ Squash Tacos or the Raw Lasagna, which are both bursting with flavors that I've yet to match with their meat rivals.

Mixed Vegetable Frittata

When I was developing this recipe, I set myself two criteria: to max out on plant-based diversity and to make it so tasty that even kids come back for seconds. This one boasts twenty-one different plant-based ingredients and the "more" approval from my two-year-old nephew—mission accomplished.

½ cup (65 g) banana flour (see Note)

½ cup (65 g) whole-grain spelt flour

½ cup (55 g) rolled oats

1 teaspoon baking powder

1 teaspoon smoked paprika

Pinch of salt

6 large eggs

¼ cup plus 1 tablespoon (70 ml) olive oil

2 zucchini, grated (3 cups/340 g)

½ large sweet potato (about 4.5 ounces/130 g), grated

1 onion, diced

2 cups (150 g) mixed sliced stir-fry vegetables (e.g., cabbage, carrot, mushroom, sprouts)

Scant ½ cup (80 g) drained and rinsed canned chickpeas

⅓ cup (65 g) drained and rinsed canned lentils

¼ cup (40 g) capers

Fresh parsley, chopped (optional)

1 medium tomato, sliced (optional)

⅓ cup (50 g) crumbled feta (optional)

2 tablespoons mixed seeds, such as flaxseed, sunflower, pumpkin, and sesame (optional)

1 teaspoon red pepper flakes (optional)

1. Preheat the oven to 375°F (190°C). Grease a 12-inch (30 cm) cake pan.

2. In a large mixing bowl, combine the banana flour, spelt flour, oats, baking powder, paprika, and salt.

3. In a separate bowl, whisk together the eggs and oil with an electric mixer until light and fluffy on top. Add the zucchini, sweet potato, onion, mixed vegetables, chickpeas, lentils, capers, and parsley, if using. Fold in the flour mixture.

4. Pour the mixture into the prepared pan. If desired, top with tomato, dot with the feta, and sprinkle with seeds and red pepper flakes.

5. Pop in the oven for 45 to 50 minutes, until cooked through. Allow to cool for 5 minutes in the pan before turning out onto a wire rack to cool completely.

> NOTE: *Banana flour is a great source of gut-loving resistant starch and is oh so tasty, but if you don't have any, replace with ¾ cup (90 g) all-purpose flour.*

Imperfection is in, perfection is out. Plants produce phytochemicals in response to stress. This is thought to be why some "ugly" fruit and vegetables, which have been subject to more stress, contain more phytochemicals. This is a great recipe to use up any stressed or bruised vegetables.

Mix-and-Match Sliders

Select one ingredient per box. Use the portions as just a guide—it's your lunch, after all.

1. Cook the items as described or according to package instructions. Grill foods with a drizzle of olive oil.

2. Assemble the ingredients according to your chosen whole-grain "plate":
   A. Wraps: Starting with any spreads, place all the ingredients on the wrap, roll, slice, and serve.
   B. Crackers: Build an open sandwich and make a side salad with the leftovers.

Whole-Grain Plate
- Wrap
- Seedy Oatcakes (page 267)
- Cheesy Vegan Crackers (page 269)
- Spiced Chickpea and Sesame Seed Crackers (page 269)
- Sourdough Wrap (page 299)

Fiber Base
(1 cup total)
- Zucchini (grilled) + butternut squash (sliced thin, grilled)
- Mixed greens + tomato (sliced)
- Alfalfa sprouts (see page 304) + radishes (sliced)
- Peppers (grilled) + arugula
- Bean sprouts + Swiss chard (steamed)

Prebiotic Boost
(to taste)
- Pomegranate seeds
- Beets (grated)
- Fennel bulb (sliced)
- Asparagus (grilled)
- Savoy cabbage (shredded)

Protein Punch
(about 2 ounces/ 50 to 70 g)
- Classic Hummus (page 264; ¼ cup)
- Tofu of choice (firm, silken, or smoked, then grilled)
- Eggs (boiled; 1 large)
- White meat of choice (chicken, turkey, pork; grilled; ⅓ cup diced)
- Legume of choice (e.g., split or green lentils; cooked; ¼ cup)

Live Kick
(1 to 2 tablespoons)
- Probiotic Yogurt (page 306)
- Aged cheese
- Raw Slaw (page 294)
- Olives
- Kimchi (page 296)

Healthy Fats
(1 tablespoon)
- Pine nuts
- Avocado
- Cashew Cheese (page 237)
- Sprinkle of mixed seeds, such as flaxseed, sunflower, pumpkin, and sesame
- Walnuts

Flavor Kick
(stir together)
- Smoked paprika (pinch) + extra virgin olive oil (1½ teaspoons)
- Apple cider vinegar (½ teaspoon) + balsamic vinegar (½ teaspoon) + extra virgin olive oil (1½ teaspoons) + fresh ground black pepper
- Lemon juice (1 tablespoon) + extra virgin olive oil (1½ tablespoon) + fresh ground black pepper
- Spinach and Walnut Pesto (page 237; 1 tablespoon)
- Natural yogurt (¼ cup/60g) + whole mustard seeds (2 teaspoons)

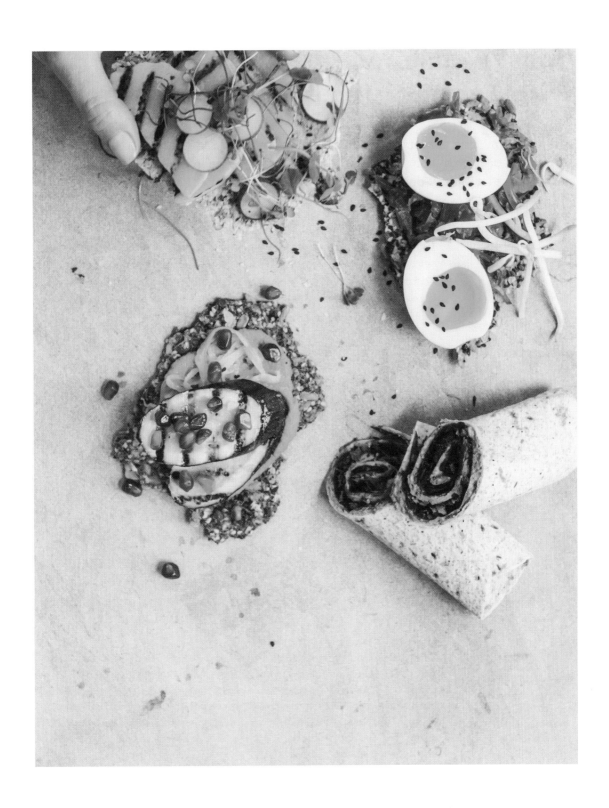

Pearl Couscous in Endive Boats with Tzatziki Dressing

Inspired by my love of *pintxos* (Basque for "snacks") and Mediterranean flavors, this is my go-to dish when I have friends over for lunch. I've been asked for the recipe so many times that I finally decided to write it down.

Endive Boats
1 teaspoon olive oil
½ cup (75 g) pearl couscous or grain of choice
1¼ cups (300 ml) boiling water
Salt
1⅓ cups (200 g) cherry tomatoes, halved
¼ red onion, sliced
1 cup (200 g) drained and rinsed canned chickpeas
¼ cup (50 g) pomegranate seeds
¼ cup (50 g) artichoke hearts, grilled and chopped
¼ cup (25 g) walnuts, chopped
¼ cup (35 g) pitted kalamata olives
9 baby mozzarella balls or scant ½ cup (60 g) crumbled feta
3.5 ounces (100 g) smoked fish of choice, roughly chopped (optional)
Fresh ground black pepper
1 large endive or little gem lettuce, divided into leaves

Tzatziki Dressing
½ cup (120 g) Probiotic Yogurt (page 306)
¼ cucumber, grated or diced
1 teaspoon olive oil
1 garlic clove, crushed
1 tablespoon fresh mint, finely sliced
Pinch of salt

1. To make the endive boats, warm the oil in a small saucepan over medium heat, then add the couscous and sauté for 3 minutes, or until golden brown. Add the boiling water and a pinch of salt and cook according to package instructions (typically 8 to 10 minutes). When al dente, drain and set aside to cool. Place in the fridge to cool completely.

2. Place the tomatoes, onion, chickpeas, pomegranate seeds, artichoke hearts, walnuts, olives, cheese, and fish, if using, in a large bowl. Stir to combine, then add the cooled couscous. Season to taste with salt and pepper.

3. To make the dressing, combine the ingredients in a small bowl. Taste and adjust the seasoning, if necessary.

4. Layer each endive "boat" with a dollop of dressing, then scoop in the couscous mix.

VARIATIONS

- Looking to expand your grain diversity? Replace half the couscous with barley.
- Craving more creaminess? Layer some Classic Hummus (page 264) on top of the tzatziki.

Couscous cooked al dente, which means "to the tooth," or to be firm to bite, not only tastes better but contains more resistant starch, a type of fiber that your GM love. This recipe further boosts the resistant starch in the dish because the couscous is served cold. Just like potato, cooking and cooling couscous increases its resistant starch. This recipe is also loaded with fructans, a type of GM-loving probiotic, from the artichoke hearts, red onion, and pomegranate seeds.

Raw Lasagna

I often get asked whether it's best to eat vegetables raw or cooked. As you guys have probably realized by now, nutrition is never black and white. Take tomatoes, for example. Cooking can destroy some nutrients (such as vitamin C), but it increases the availability of other beneficial phytochemicals (such as lycopene, which is linked with skin health). The best thing is to mix it up: Sometimes go raw, sometimes go cooked. Here's a tasty raw lasagna to get you started.

Cashew Cheese
1 cup (140 g) cashews
1½ cups (120 ml) warm water
2½ tablespoons nutritional yeast
1 tablespoon fresh lemon juice
2 garlic cloves
1½ teaspoons Dijon mustard
Pinch of salt

Spinach and Walnut Pesto
2⅔ cups (40 g) basil leaves, plus extra for garnish
1⅓ cups (40 g) spinach
½ cup (50 g) walnuts
2 teaspoons fresh lemon juice
1 garlic clove
1½ tablespoons nutritional yeast
2 tablespoons extra virgin olive oil
Pinch of salt

Lasagna
2 large zucchini
4 medium tomatoes, thinly sliced

Cherry tomatoes (optional)
Fresh ground black pepper

1. To make the cashew cheese, place all the ingredients in a blender. Blend for 2 to 3 minutes until smooth. Taste and adjust salt as needed. Set aside.

2. To make the pesto, rinse the blender with water, then add all the ingredients. Blend until everything is combined to your preferred texture. You may need to scrape down any mixture that has risen up the sides a few times. Add a dash more oil, if needed.

3. To assemble the lasagna, slice the zucchini into thin strips using a mandoline or peeler.

4. On each serving plate, place a few slices of zucchini, followed by the cashew cheese, tomato slices, and, finally, pesto. Repeat the layering, starting with the zucchini. Aim for two to three layers, finishing with the cashew cheese on top. Garnish with extra basil leaves, cherry tomatoes, if using, and pepper to serve.

VARIATION

 • If you have your own favorite lasagna recipe, why not switch some of the dairy cheese for this plant-based cashew version?

Leafy greens, including spinach and basil, are a great source of the phytochemicals lutein and zeaxanthin. Not only are these widely recognized as important for eye health, but in a trial they've also been shown to improve how quickly our brains process what we're seeing.[1] This suggests they might help prevent the decline in our brain function as we age.

Sautéed Brussels Sprouts and Broccolini with Pesto and Wild Rice

Whoever thinks *greens* means boring needs to try this. Full of prebiotics, this cruciferous duo is good enough to convert any anti-greens advocate. It also boasts close to 8 grams of fiber per portion and will have their GM singing out for seconds.

Pesto
1⅔ cups (40 g) basil
2 tablespoons pine nuts
2 tablespoons chopped walnuts
¼ cup (60 ml) extra virgin olive oil
2 tablespoons grated Parmesan
1 garlic clove
Salt

Rice and Vegetables
1 cup (150 g) wild rice or grain(s) of choice
1 tablespoon extra virgin olive oil
2 garlic cloves, chopped
10 ounces (280 g) firm tofu, or protein of choice, cut into strips
9 ounces (250 g) mushrooms, halved
7 ounces (200 g) broccolini, quartered
1⅓ cups (125 g) brussels sprouts, halved

1. To make the pesto, place all the ingredients in a food processor and pulse until combined to your preferred texture. You may need to scrape down any mixture that has risen up the sides a few times.

2. To make the rice and vegetables, cook the rice according to the package instructions.

3. Warm a frying pan over medium heat and add the oil and garlic. Fry for 1 to 2 minutes, then add the tofu. Fry on both sides for 5 minutes, or until golden brown. Remove from the pan.

4. Place the mushrooms, broccolini, sprouts, and 2 tablespoons water in the same pan. Sauté until tender, about 5 minutes.

5. Remove from the heat, then add the tofu back in and stir in the pesto to warm.

6. Plate the warm rice and top with the tofu and vegetables.

VARIATION

* If you're not a fan of sprouts or broccoli, swap them out for your favorite vegetables.

In terms of health benefits, extra virgin olive oil (EVOO) is hands down the superior oil option. Loaded with polyphenols and other phytochemicals, the wide-ranging health benefits, including heart, brain, and gut health, are supported by several trials.[2] You can also cook with it, despite the myths. High-quality EVOO has a high smoke point (around 400°F/200°C), and research has shown that it's comparatively stable during home cooking, thanks to its high-antioxidant capacity, which protects the fat.[3]

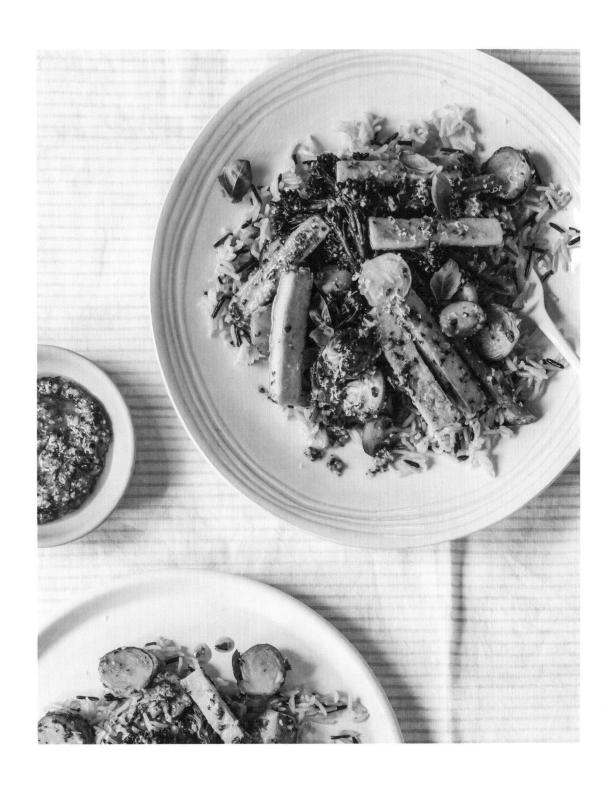

Korean BBQ Squash Tacos with Kimchi

A showcase of fermented-food flavors—just another reason to be grateful for our microbial friends. Gochujang, a Korean fermented red chili paste, and kimchi, a Korean fermented-cabbage side dish, are the perfect foods, owing to the winning combination of flavors and attributed health benefits. With close to 10 grams of fiber per portion, this is one dish you have to try! While the squash marinates, try the Do-Nothing Exercise (see page 180).

1 medium butternut squash, seeded, peeled, and quartered (see Notes)
3 garlic cloves, minced
3 scallions, sliced
2 tablespoons tamari or soy sauce
1½ tablespoons gochujang (see Notes)
1 tablespoon sesame oil
1 Medjool date, crushed into a paste with 1 tablespoon boiling water
Fresh ground black pepper
4 whole wheat tortillas (or Sourdough Wraps, page 299)

Toppings
2 tomatoes, diced
⅓ cup (50 g) Kimchi (page 296)
¼ cup (60 g) Probiotic Yogurt (page 306)
1 avocado, sliced
1 handful cilantro, chopped
2 tablespoons sesame seeds (optional)

1. Preheat the oven to 375°F (190°C).

2. Grate the squash, using a food processor or box grater. (See Notes if you're in a hurry.)

3. Place the garlic, scallions, tamari, gochujang, oil, date paste, and pepper in a large bowl and mix well. Stir in the squash, making sure everything is coated. Leave to marinate for 20 minutes while you prepare the toppings.

4. Spread the marinated squash on a baking sheet. Bake in the oven for 15 minutes before giving it a quick mix. Return to the oven for 5 more minutes, or until caramelized on the outside.

5. Meanwhile, place a baking rack over a baking pan and drape each tortilla on the rack, forming hard taco shells. Place in the oven, with the squash, for the final 10 to 15 minutes.

6. Allow the taco shells to cool before filling each with a spoonful of the warm squash, then top with all the good stuff: tomatoes, kimchi, yogurt, avocado, cilantro, and sesame seeds, if using.

> NOTES:
>
> • *Short on time? Steam the squash in the microwave for 5 minutes before coating in the marinade and browning in the oven for a final 10 minutes.*
>
> • *Want to really impress your friends? Replace the squash with jackfruit.*
>
> • *Sensitive to spicy food? Halve the quantity of gochujang, which is available online or in most Asian grocers.*

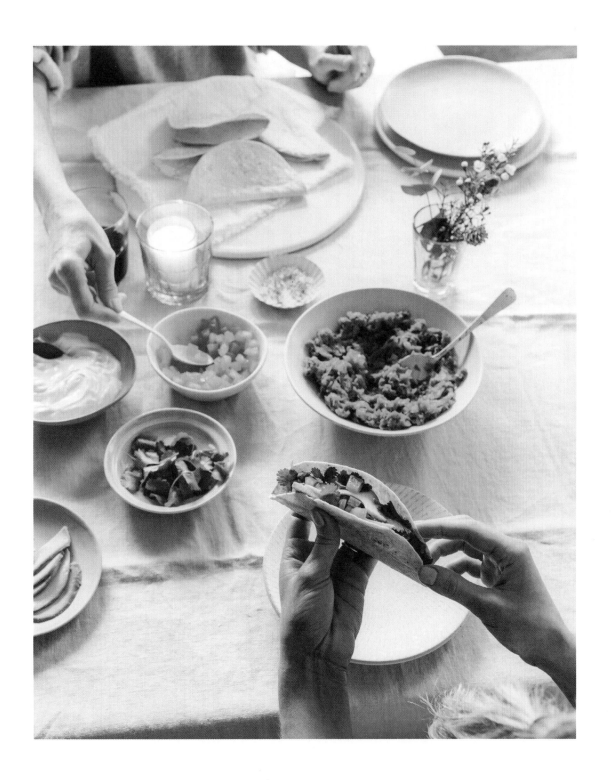

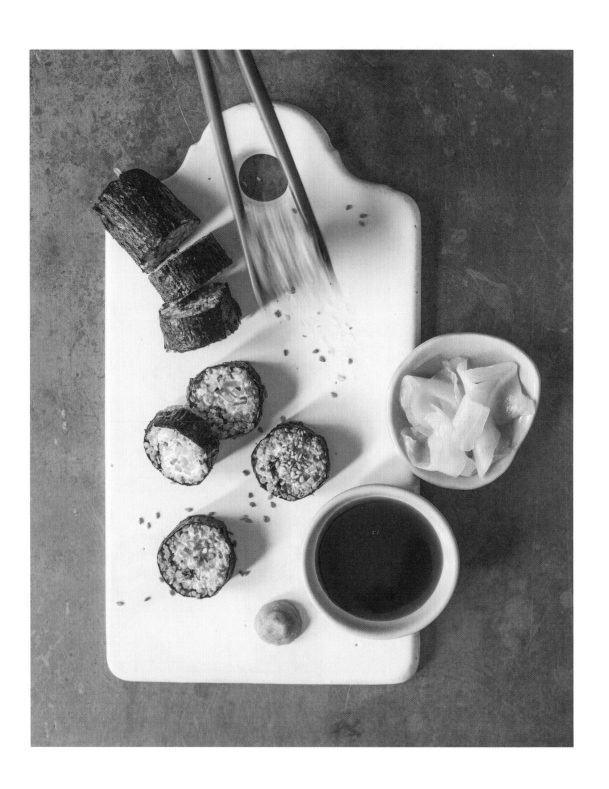

Quinoa Sushi Rolls

With double the fiber of store-bought sushi, this is a high-protein, fiber-boosted tweak on my childhood favorite. I also added red onion, which is an especially good source of the polyphenol quercetin, known for its antioxidant benefits.

1 teaspoon white miso paste
1 tablespoon ground flaxseed
1 tablespoon hot water
⅔ cup (120 g) cooked quinoa
2 nori sheets
2 tablespoons Probiotic
   Yogurt (page 306)
½ carrot, julienned
½ cucumber, julienned
½ red bell pepper, julienned
⅛ red onion, julienned
½ avocado, sliced
2 ounces (60 g) smoked
   salmon (or protein of
   choice), sliced

Extras
Sesame seeds
Pickled ginger or Raw Slaw
   (page 294)
Light soy sauce, or dipping
   sauce of choice

1. Place the miso, flaxseed, and hot water into a small mug and stir to combine, then pour it over the quinoa and stir through. Place in the fridge for 10 minutes to thicken.

2. Cover a bamboo sushi rolling mat (or folded kitchen cloth) with a large piece of plastic wrap. Place a nori sheet on top of the mat and spread ⅓ cup (60 g) of the quinoa across three quarters of the nori sheet. Leave a quarter of the nori roll free to help seal it (step 5). Press the quinoa firmly into the mat using the bottom of a cup.

3. Spread 1 tablespoon of the yogurt over the quinoa, 2 inches (5 cm) in from the edge.

4. Lay half of the strips of carrot, cucumber, pepper, onion, avocado, and salmon, if using, on top of the yogurt.

5. To roll, start with the edge closest to the filling. Tightly roll the end over the filling, pressing as you go. Press the edges together at the end, using a tiny bit of water on the sheet's edge to help seal it.

6. With a sharp knife, cut into pieces, then sprinkle with sesame seeds. Repeat with the other nori sheet and the remaining ingredients, then serve with pickles and a dipping sauce.

VARIATION

* The filling options are endless—experiment with your favorite flavors. Try replacing the cucumber with sugar snap peas.

Regular consumption of seaweed has been shown to modify your GM's genetic potential, meaning they develop the ability to digest parts of the seaweed. This is something that an untrained GM can't do. A GM with more skills: Sign me up!

Dinner

No matter what sort of day you've had, I'm a firm believer that dinner shouldn't add to your worries. If you're looking for convenience, you'll find the Mix-and-Match Gut-Goodness Bowls, which are all about laying down the foundation for a DIY throw-together dish that doesn't fall short on taste or diversity. For those Friday-night cravings, you'll find pizza duos and a spicy bean burger with options to match everyone's nutritional needs and flavor requests. What about the meat lovers? Even they'll be singing your praises when they try the meatless meatballs in rich tomato sauce and the meaty lentil and mushroom fettuccine.

Butter Bean Curry in a Butternut Squash Bowl

This rich, creamy curry, served in an edible bowl of roasted butternut squash, really does symbolize the idea of "comfort in a bowl." It's also loaded with vitamins A, K, and C, making it quite nourishing. Short on time? Don't let that put you off. Ditch the edible bowl and just go for the curry—it's one of my winter staples.

Butternut Squash Bowl

2 small butternut squash (each about 1 pound/450 g), halved lengthwise and seeded

1 teaspoon olive oil

Butter Bean Curry

2 teaspoons olive oil

½ onion, finely chopped

1 garlic clove, sliced

1½ tablespoons grated fresh ginger

2 tablespoons Thai red curry paste

1 teaspoon curry powder

One 15-ounce (425 g) can butter beans, drained and rinsed

One 13.5-ounce (400 ml) can coconut milk

Half a 14.5-ounce (411 g) can diced tomatoes

3 to 5 ounces (about 80 to 150 g) leafy greens such as bok choy and spinach

7 ounces (200 g) boneless white fish of choice (optional)

1 cup (15 g) cilantro, finely chopped

⅔ cup (100 g) frozen peas

2 tablespoons tamari or soy sauce

Salt

Fresh ground black pepper

Fresh lime juice

1. To make the squash bowl, preheat the oven to 400°F (200°C). Line a baking sheet with parchment paper.

2. Place the squash in a microwave-safe dish with a little water in the bottom, cover, and cook on high for 15 minutes, or until soft. Allow to cool before scooping out the flesh with a spoon, leaving the sides of the squash "bowl" about 2 cm thick. Set aside 2 cups (400 g) of the flesh for the curry.

3. Place the squash bowls on the prepared baking sheet and massage the oil into the flesh and skin. Bake for 20 minutes, or until golden brown.

4. To make the curry, warm a large frying pan over high heat, add the oil, onion, garlic, ginger, curry paste, and curry powder, and stir for 2 to 3 minutes, until fragrant.

5. Add the beans, coconut milk, tomatoes, and squash flesh. Reduce the heat to a gentle simmer and cook for 10 to 15 minutes until the squash is fork-tender.

3. Add your leafy greens and fish, if using, and continue stirring for 3 minutes, or until the greens (and fish) are almost cooked.

4. Add the cilantro, peas, and tamari. Taste and adjust the seasoning. Once the peas are cooked and the greens still have a little bit of crunch to them, remove from the heat.

5. Squeeze in lime juice to taste, spoon into the squash bowl, and serve warm.

The claims around ginger being a remedy for indigestion and nausea are backed by science. How? Trials have shown that ginger, albeit at fairly high doses, can speed up the emptying of food from your stomach into your small intestine.[4]

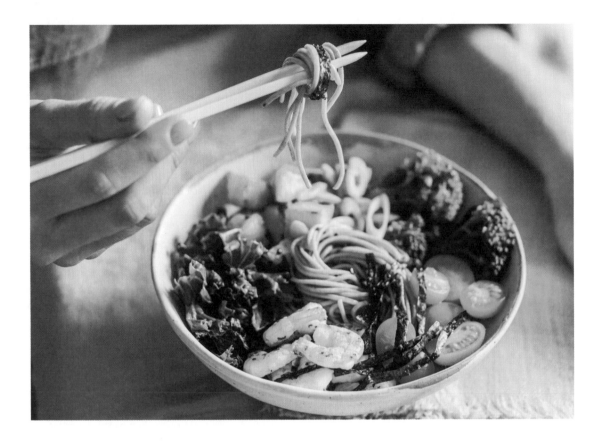

Mix-and-Match
Gut-Goodness Bowls

Select one column of
ingredients or create your
own combo by picking one
ingredient per row.

1. Cook the items as described. (Grill foods with a drizzle of
olive oil. Steam in a pot or microwave.) Prepare your grains
according to package instructions.

2. Combine dressing ingredients.

3. Assemble your bowl and finish with dressing.

	Monday	**Tuesday**	**Wednesday**	**Thursday**	**Friday**
Fiber Base (about 2 cups raw)	Peas Cauliflower (steamed)	Sweet potato (steamed) Onion (sliced and fried)	Kale (steamed)	Broccoli (steamed) Sugar snap peas	Zucchini ribbons (grilled)
Golden Grains (3 to 4 oz/80 to 120 g cooked)	Wild or brown rice (½ to ¾ cup)	Buckwheat soba noodles (¾ to 1 cup)	Quinoa (½ to ⅔ cup)	Wheat berries (⅓ to ½ cup)	Whole grain pasta (¾ to 1 cup)
Polyphenol Hit (½ cup raw)	Red bell pepper Cilantro (1 tablespoon)	Baby spinach	Sweet corn	1 nori sheet (torn into strips)	Cherry tomatoes
Fermented Flavors (1 to 2 tablespoons)	Kimchi (page 296)	Raw Slaw (page 294)	Probiotic Yogurt (page 306)	Pickles	Shaved Parmesan
Prebiotic Boost (to taste)	Banana (sliced)	Asparagus (grilled)	Chopped scallion	Savoy cabbage	Brussels sprouts (grilled)
Healthy Fats (1 tablespoon)	Cashews	Pumpkin seeds	Avocado	Sesame seeds	Walnuts
Protein Punch (3 to 4 oz/80 to 120 g)	Chicken breast (cooked, ⅔ to ¾ cup diced)	Tofu (firm, ⅓ to ½ cup)	Two eggs (boiled or fried)	Seafood of choice (mackerel, salmon, shrimp, squid; cooked)	White beans (cooked from dry; or rinsed, drained, and warmed; canned; ½ to ⅔ cup)
Dressing (1 to 2 tablespoons; adjust to taste, including a pinch of salt)	**Red Curry** Thai red curry paste (2 teaspoons)* Probiotic Yogurt (¼ cup/60 g; page 306) Unsweetened shredded coconut (2 teaspoons)	**Whole-Grain Mustard** Whole-grain mustard (1 teaspoon) Olive oil (1½ teaspoons)	**Hot Sauce** Sriracha (½ teaspoon) Minced fresh ginger (1 teaspoon) Apple cider vinegar (½ teaspoon)	**Miso Sauce** White miso paste (1 teaspoon) Probiotic Yogurt (¼ cup/60 g; page 306)	**Basil Dressing** Extra virgin olive oil (1½ teaspoons) Lemon juice (1 teaspoon) 4 basil leaves (finely chopped)

Use this to coat the protein, along with a brush of olive oil, before grilling.

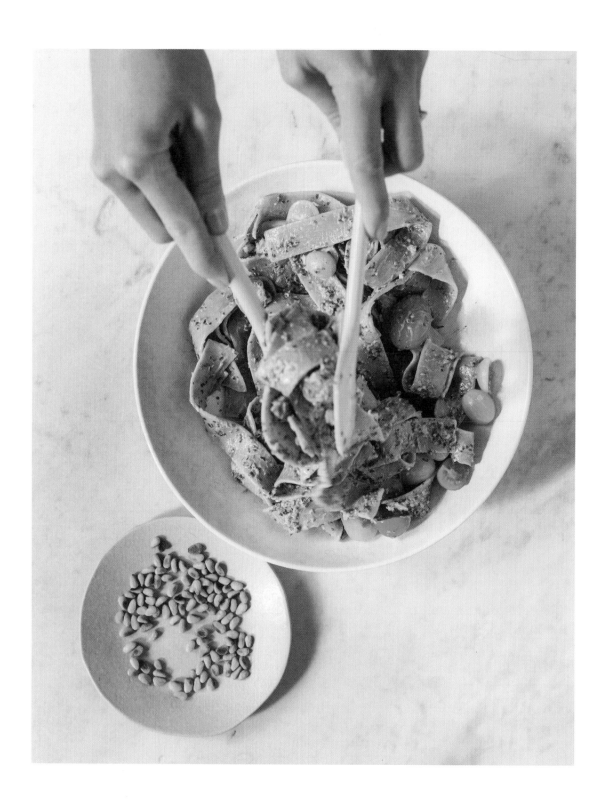

Creamy Pistachio and Spinach Pesto Pasta

For those nightmare days when all you want is something quick and tasty. And don't worry, it's got your microbes covered, too, with the prebiotic pistachios and 9 grams of fiber per portion—it's a real GM favorite.

Pesto

3 ounces (80 g) spinach
Scant 1 cup (20 g) basil
   leaves
½ cup (65 g) pistachios
½ avocado
Scant ½ cup (100 g)
   Probiotic Yogurt
   (page 306)
1 garlic clove
3 tablespoons nutritional
   yeast
2 tablespoons extra virgin
   olive oil
2 teaspoons fresh lemon
   juice
Pinch of salt

Pasta

7 ounces (200 g) whole grain
   pasta of choice

Extras

1 pint (10 ounces/300 g)
   cherry tomatoes, halved
2 tablespoons pine nuts
   (optional)
Fresh ground black pepper

1. Place all the pesto ingredients into a blender along with 2 tablespoons water. Pulse to combine to your preferred texture. You may need to scrape down any mixture that has risen up the sides a few times.

2. Cook the pasta according to the package instructions, then coat with the pesto and leave for 5 minutes to infuse.

3. Serve topped with cherry tomatoes and pine nuts, if using, and some fresh ground black pepper.

VARIATION

◆ Replace the nutritional yeast with ⅓ cup (35 g) freshly grated Pecorino Romano or Parmesan cheese.

It's worth paying a bit extra for extra virgin olive oil. Making EVOO is an expensive process. While a higher price doesn't always ensure quality, the cheapest bottle on the shelf is unlikely to be the real thing. To save on cost, I buy in bulk and decant a portion into a dark bottle (which protects it from sunlight), as I use it in all my cooking.

Satay Tofu Skewers
with Saucy Greens

I grew up in Queensland, Australia, where alfresco dining happens all year round. These skewers remind me of home, of sitting around the table watching them sizzle away on the barbecue. With chewy grains and tender greens, this dish is high in protein and will bring you half your daily fiber needs.

Satay Tofu
3 tablespoons sriracha
2 tablespoons tamari or soy sauce
1 tablespoon sesame oil
½ Medjool date, softened, or sweetener of choice
1 teaspoon peanut butter
½ teaspoon garlic powder
10 ounces (280 g) firm tofu, cut into 1½-inch (4 cm) cubes
1 red bell pepper, cut into 1½-inch (4 cm) squares
1 green or red bell pepper, cut into 1½-inch (4 cm) squares

Saucy Greens
1 teaspoon sesame oil
2 garlic cloves, sliced
21 ounces (600 g) mixed greens such as kale, chard, bok choy, sliced
1⅔ cups (400 g) cooked wheat berries, or other cooked grain of choice
Tamari or soy sauce, to taste
Salt
Freshly ground black pepper

Dipping Sauce
Probiotic Yogurt (optional; page 306)

1. To make the satay tofu, place the sriracha, tamari, oil, date, peanut butter, and garlic powder in a large bowl and mix well. Stir in the tofu and leave to marinate for at least 1 hour. Prepare the grill if barbecuing.

2. Skewer the tofu, alternating with the peppers. Set aside any leftover marinade.

3. Place the skewers on the grill or a griddle pan over medium heat. Char on each side, then lower the heat and cook through, approximately 2 minutes on each side. Cover and remove from the the heat.

4. To make the greens, warm a large frying pan over high heat and add the oil and garlic. Cook for 1 to 2 minutes, then add the greens and wheat berries. Stir-fry for 2 to 3 minutes, until the greens have wilted. Remove from the heat, drizzle on the tamari, and season to taste.

5. Serve the stir-fry topped with the skewers and a side of remaining marinade or yogurt for dipping.

VARIATIONS

* Try replacing the grains with lentils for a higher prebiotic punch.

* Short on time? Replace the satay sauce with ¼ cup (70 g) peanut butter, 2 teaspoons curry powder, and ⅓ cup plus 1 tablespoon (100 ml) coconut milk.

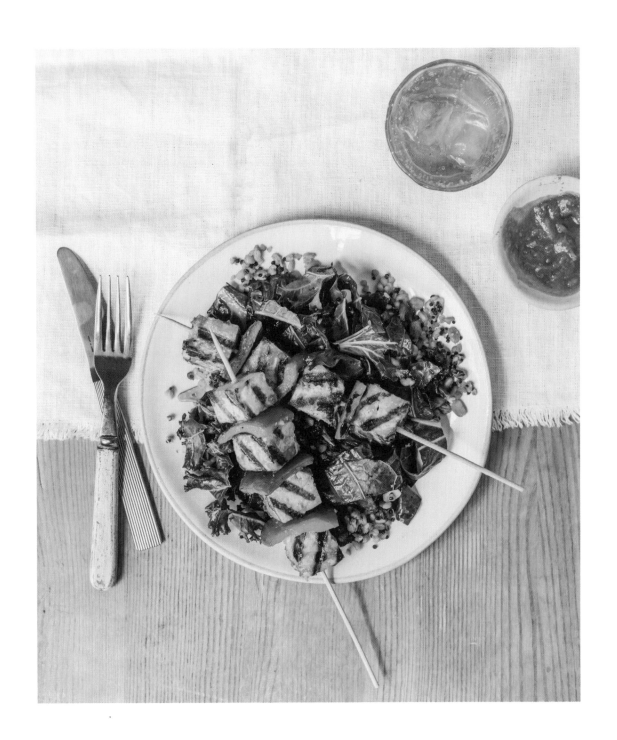

Eggplant Cannelloni with Beet Salsa and Cashew Cheese

Looking for that wow factor? Then this dish is for you! The compliments won't stop on presentation—the creamy cashew cheese matched with the zesty salsa and succulent eggplant makes it one to remember.

Oil, for greasing
2 eggplants (about 21 ounces/600g)
Cashew Cheese (page 237)

Beet Salsa
14 ounces (400 g) cooked beets in vinegar or pickled beets (about 8 medium)
8 cherry tomatoes
1¼ cups (20 g) cilantro leaves, plus extra for garnish
2 teaspoons fresh lemon juice
1 teaspoon red pepper flakes
2 tablespoons extra virgin olive oil
Salt
Fresh ground black pepper

Olive Pesto
¼ cup (30 g) crumbled feta
2 tablespoons extra virgin olive oil
¼ cup (45 g) pitted kalamata olives
⅔ cup (115 g) drained and rinsed canned cannellini beans

1. Preheat the oven to 375°F (190°C). Grease a 9 × 13 (23 × 33 cm) baking dish.

2. Slice the eggplant lengthwise into thin sheets about ½ inch (1 cm) thick.

3. Grease a griddle pan and warm over medium-high heat, then add the eggplant and grill for 5 minutes on each side, or until cooked through.

4. Meanwhile, place the beet salsa ingredients in a blender and combine roughly. Set aside.

5. Rinse the blender with water, then place the pesto ingredients in it and blend to a coarse consistency.

6. To assemble the cannelloni, lay out the grilled eggplant strips, layer each one with some of the cashew cheese and pesto, then top with a little of the salsa, roll up, and place in the prepared baking dish.

7. Bake in the oven for 15 minutes, or until the flavors have cooked through and the tops are golden brown.

8. To serve, spread a spoonful of the salsa on each plate and add the stuffed cannelloni. Top with a little more salsa and cilantro leaves.

Beets are a great source of nitrates, which are Mother Nature's alternative to medications for lowering blood pressure. In fact, there are several trials showing a benefit in people with high blood pressure.[5]

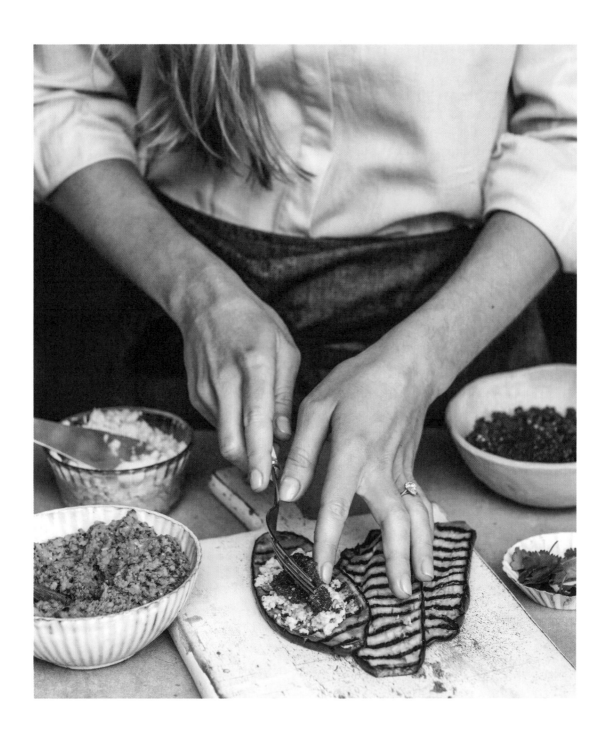

Pizza Duo

It's all about the crust—thin and crispy. Pizza is such a fun, versatile meal, and it can be easily adapted to accommodate both your and your microbes' nutritional needs and taste preferences—it's one that everyone can enjoy. Here are two of my favorites, boasting over 10 grams of fiber per portion.

Spelt and Quinoa

Crust
1 cup (120 g) whole-grain spelt flour, plus extra for kneading
2 teaspoons baking powder
1 teaspoon Italian seasoning
Pinch of salt
¼ cup (50 g) cooked quinoa
½ cup (120 g) Greek yogurt
1½ tablespoons extra virgin olive oil

Pizza Sauce
1 cup (150 g) cherry tomatoes
2 tablespoons chopped basil
6 sun-dried tomatoes, preserved in oil
1 garlic clove
1 tablespoon olive oil

Topping Inspo
Pick one combination or add your own favorites
Sautéed mushrooms + spinach + goat cheese
Roasted peppers + arugula + pine nuts
Kalamata olives + grilled artichoke hearts + ricotta cheese

1. Preheat the oven to 400°F (200°C).

2. To make the pizza crust, combine the flour, baking powder, Italian seasoning, and salt in a large bowl, then stir in the quinoa and fold in the yogurt. Using your hands, form a wet dough. Knead on a floured surface for 3 to 4 minutes, rolling into a ball, then flattening out (think of it as yoga for your pizza dough). Separate into two balls before placing in a bowl and coating with the oil. Cover with an inverted bowl and leave to sit somewhere warm for 15 minutes.

3. Place the rested dough on a clean work surface and, using your hands, spread it out to form your pizza crust. Pinch the edge to form a crust.

4. Bake for 10 minutes, or until slightly golden, ideally on a perforated baking sheet, so the pizza crust gets nice and crispy.

5. While the crust cooks, make the pizza sauce. Place the cherry tomatoes, basil, sun-dried tomatoes, garlic, and oil in a blender and pulse roughly.

6. Remove the crust from the oven, then spread with the pizza sauce and add other toppings. Bake for an additional 5 to 10 minutes, depending on your toppings.

7. Slice and serve.

VARIATIONS

* Prefer to keep your hands clean? Use a Spelt Wrap (see page 271) as your crust.

* Replace the spices with fresh herbs of your choice, like oregano or basil.

Buckwheat and Oat

Short on time? No oven required for this crust! All it needs is 5 minutes in the frying pan, and your low-FODMAP pizza is ready.

Crust
⅓ cup plus 1½ tablespoons (70 g) buckwheat groats
½ cup (40 g) rolled oats
1½ teaspoons olive oil, plus extra for frying
1 large egg
1 teaspoon baking powder
Pinch of salt

Low-FODMAP Pizza Sauce
1 cup (150 g) cherry tomatoes
2 tablespoons chopped basil
6 sun-dried tomatoes, preserved in oil
1 tablespoon garlic-infused olive oil

Topping Inspo
Pick one combination or add your own favorites
Classic Hummus (page 264) + roasted peppers + plum tomatoes
Ricotta cheese + roasted butternut squash + caramelized red onion
Tahini Dressing (page 256) + smoked salmon + spinach + sauerkraut

Low-FODMAP Topping Inspo
Roasted eggplant + green olives + feta
BBQ chicken + roasted peppers + mozzarella
Kalamata olives + Parmesan + arugula

1. To make the crust, place the buckwheat, oats, oil, egg, baking powder, and salt in a blender along with ¾ cup plus 1 tablespoon (200 ml) water and blend for 30 seconds.

2. Warm a little oil in a nonstick frying pan over medium heat. Pour ⅓ cup (75 ml) of the batter into the pan to form a mini pizza.

3. Cook for about 3 minutes, until there are bubbles in the base and you can lift it to flip easily.

4. Turn the heat down and spread on the sauce and toppings of choice. Place a lid or another pan over the top to seal in the heat. Cook for another 2 to 3 minutes, or until the toppings are done to your liking. Transfer to a plate and cover to keep warm.

5. Repeat with the remaining batter.

Grilled Miso Eggplant
with Sweet Potato Wedges

Serves 2

A meaty dish that marries a succulent fillet of marinated eggplant with crispy-skinned potato wedges. This high-fiber dish wouldn't be complete without the creamy tahini dressing, which is so tasty I always make a double batch for my Gut-Goodness Bowls (page 246).

Miso Marinade
1½ tablespoons white miso paste
1 garlic clove, crushed
2 teaspoons sesame oil
½ Medjool date, stirred into a paste with 1 tablespoon hot water

Tahini Dressing
1 tablespoon tahini
1 tablespoon extra virgin olive oil
Juice of ½ a lemon
½ garlic clove, crushed
Salt
Fresh ground black pepper

Grilled Eggplant
Olive oil, for greasing
1 large eggplant, cut lengthwise into 4 slices

Roasted Vegetables
1 large sweet potato (about 10 ounces/300 g), cut into thin wedges
2 teaspoons olive oil
1 cup (150 g) cherry tomatoes
Salt
Fresh ground black pepper

Extras
Side salad of arugula or greens of choice

1. Preheat the oven to 375°F (190°C). Line a baking sheet with parchment paper.

2. To make the miso marinade, combine the miso paste, garlic, sesame oil, and date paste in a small bowl with 1 tablespoon water.

3. To make the tahini dressing, combine the tahini, extra virgin olive oil, lemon juice, and garlic in a small bowl with 1 tablespoon water. Season to taste.

4. To make the eggplant, grease a griddle pan over high heat, warm and grill the eggplant for 2 minutes on each side, or until brown grill marks are formed. (If you're short on time, skip this step.)

5. Transfer the eggplant to the prepared baking sheet and pour on the miso marinade. Using your hands, massage the marinade into the flesh and bake in the oven for 10 minutes.

6. To make the roasted vegetables, place the sweet potato wedges in a microwave-safe dish with a little water in the bottom, cover, and cook on high for 4 minutes to soften.

7. Pat the wedges dry, then toss them in the olive oil with the tomatoes and sprinkle with salt and pepper.

8. Add the wedges and tomatoes to the baking sheet with the eggplant and cook in the oven for an additional 15 to 20 minutes, or until crisp on the outside.

9. Serve the eggplant slices alongside the sweet potato wedges, tomatoes, and side salad. Drizzle with the tahini dressing and dig in.

Sweet potato is rich in many plant compounds, including beta-carotene, which is responsible for its orange glow. This antioxidant is transformed into vitamin A in our body to support immunity and eye health. To maximize beta-carotene absorption, I've added olive oil—the resulting crispy crunch is a bonus.

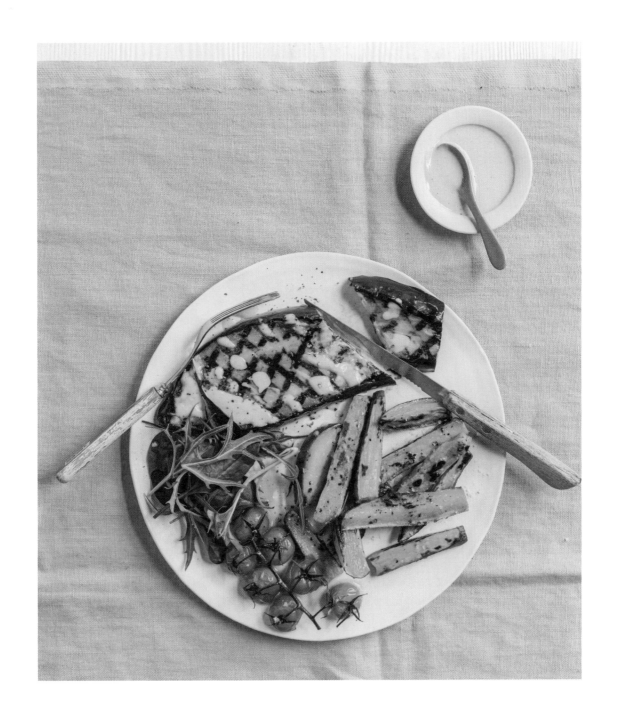

Meatless Meatballs in Rich Tomato Sauce

I might be a little biased, but my microbes and I much prefer these to the meat version—they're incredibly tender and full of flavor, and they provide 15 grams of fiber per portion.

Meatballs
1 tablespoon olive oil
1 eggplant (about
    14 ounces/400 g), diced
1 onion, chopped
1 teaspoon garlic powder
¼ cup pitted kalamata
    olives, sliced
3 sun-dried tomatoes,
    preserved in oil
2 tablespoons
    Worcestershire sauce
2 teaspoons Italian
    seasoning
Pinch of salt
½ cup (60 g) rolled oats
2 tablespoons flaxseeds
Scant ½ cup (10 g) basil

Tomato Sauce
1 teaspoon olive oil
1 garlic clove
3 sun-dried tomatoes,
    preserved in oil
Half a 14.5-ounce (411 g)
    can diced tomatoes
2 tablespoons chopped
    basil
Pinch of salt

Extras (optional)
1⅓ cups (40 g) spinach
Probiotic Yogurt (page 306)
    or Parmesan

1. Preheat the oven to 375°F (190°C). Line a baking sheet with parchment paper.

2. To make the meatballs, warm a large frying pan over medium heat, add the oil, then the eggplant, onion, garlic powder, olives, sun-dried tomatoes, Worcestershire sauce, Italian seasoning, and salt, and sauté for 5 to 10 minutes, until starting to color.

3. Place the oats and flaxseeds in a food processor and blend to form coarse crumbs. Transfer to a bowl and set aside. Place the sautéed mix, along with the basil, in the food processor. Combine roughly.

4. Transfer to the bowl with the crumb mixture, stir to combine, and leave in the fridge to thicken for 10 minutes.

5. Remove from the fridge and roll into golf ball–size "meatballs" (makes around 12) and place on the prepared baking sheet, then bake in the oven for 20 minutes, or until golden brown.

6. Meanwhile, prepare the tomato sauce. Warm a saucepan over medium heat and add the oil, garlic, and sun-dried tomatoes. Sauté for a few minutes, then add the diced tomatoes, basil, and salt. Reduce the heat to a gentle simmer and cook for about 20 minutes, stirring every few minutes.

7. Serve the meatballs on a bed of spinach, if desired, and topped with the tomato sauce and yogurt, if you like.

VARIATIONS

- Spice things up by adding half a chile to the sauce.

- For vegans: Use vegan Worcestershire sauce, or replace with barbecue sauce, and use vegan yogurt and cheese, or omit them, for serving.

Garlic has been used for its medicinal benefits for thousands of years, and now we have the science to back it up. Trials have shown that garlic can have positive effects on blood pressure and cholesterol management.[6] And what about its flu-fighting power? There have been some quality trials to support this, too.[7]

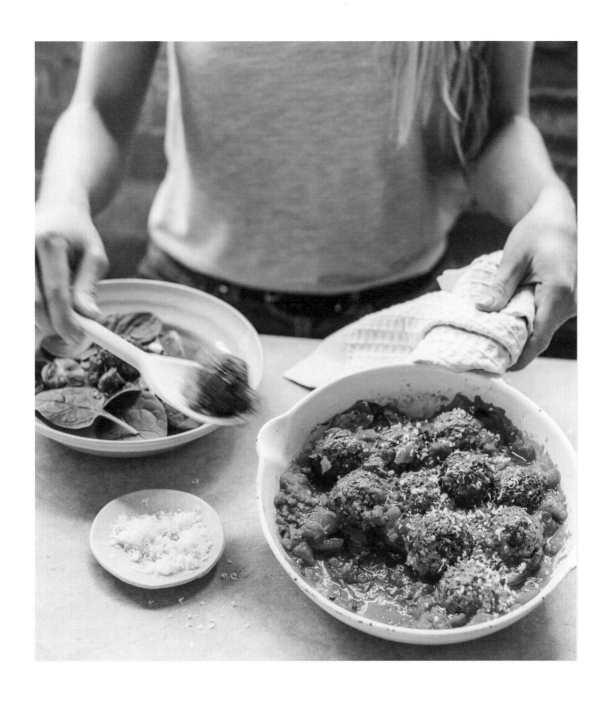

Spicy Bean Burgers

BBQs just got a whole lot tastier. With the prebiotic goodness of the legumes and polyphenols from the herbs and spices, the burger alone offers over 5 grams of fiber, making it a tasty feast for your microbes, too.

Burger Patties

½ large sweet potato (about 4.5 ounces/130 g), chopped
One 15-ounce (425 g) can mixed beans, drained and rinsed
1 scallion, chopped
1 medium carrot (about 2 ounces/60 g), grated
1 large egg
⅓ cup (10 g) fresh cilantro, chopped
1 teaspoon garlic powder
1 teaspoon ground cumin
1 teaspoon smoked paprika
1 teaspoon diced chile or red pepper flakes
1 tablespoon tamari or soy sauce
1 tablespoon fresh lime juice
Fresh ground black pepper
½ cup (40 g) rolled oats
1 teaspoon arrowroot starch
½ cup (50 g) grated cheese (optional)
½ cup (40 g) unsweetened shredded coconut

Caramelized Onions

1 red onion, cut into thin rings
½ Medjool date, diced
1 tablespoon balsamic vinegar
1 tablespoon olive oil

To Serve

Olive oil, for cooking
6 whole-grain burger buns (or go naked)
Pickled beets, sliced
Tomatoes, sliced
Probiotic Yogurt (page 306)
Classic Hummus, Pea and Mint Hummus, or Harissa Dip (pages 264 to 266)

1. To make the burger patties, place the sweet potato and a small splash of water into a microwave-safe dish. Cover and cook on high for 4 minutes. Drain and cool.

2. Combine the beans, scallion, and carrot in a large bowl. Set aside about 1 cup (130 g) of the mixture and transfer the rest to a food processor.

3. Add the egg, cilantro, garlic powder, cumin, paprika, chile, tamari, lime juice, and black pepper to the food processor. Blend roughly, then transfer to a large bowl.

4. Stir in the reserved bean mixture and the oats, arrowroot, and cheese, if using, and place in the fridge for 10 minutes to firm up.

5. Remove from the fridge, then form the mixture into six palm-size patties (about 2.5 ounces/75 g each) and gently coat with the coconut.

6. To make the caramelized onions, place the onion, date, vinegar, and oil in a small saucepan with ⅓ cup (80 ml) water and cook over low heat for 15 to 20 minutes, until soft and caramelized.

7. Warm some oil in a frying pan over medium-low heat. Add the patties and cook for 4 to 5 minutes on each side, until golden brown.

8. Finally, the burger build! Layer each bun with the beet, tomato, and a dollop of yogurt, if using, followed by the patty and caramelized onions.

Cumin is packed full of plant bioactives that are linked to improved immunity, heart health, and even digestion—it's not just a tasty addition.

Lentil and Mushroom Fettuccine

My favorite dish growing up was my Nanna's traditional fettuccine, which, although it was oh so tasty, didn't provide much goodness for my microbes. I challenged myself to make a meat-free version, with all the flavor but none of the meat. It turned out to be quite the hit—the family didn't miss the meat either. And it delivers over 50 percent of our daily fiber recommendations per portion.

1 onion, chopped
2 garlic cloves, chopped
1 celery rib, chopped
1 carrot, chopped
1 zucchini, chopped
1 red bell pepper, seeded and chopped
5 ounces (150 g) mushrooms, chopped
2 tablespoons olive oil
3 bay leaves
1 teaspoon Italian seasoning
One 15-ounce (425 g) can of green lentils, drained and rinsed
One 14.5-ounce (411 g) can whole peeled tomatoes
6 sun-dried tomatoes, preserved in oil, chopped
2 tablespoons tomato paste
2 tablespoons capers
1⅔ cups (400 ml) vegetable stock
Salt
Fresh ground black pepper
7 ounces (200 g) whole grain fettuccine
Parmesan or nutritional yeast, to serve

1. Place the onion, garlic, celery, carrot, zucchini, red pepper, and mushrooms in a blender and blend for a few seconds until finely chopped.

2. Warm a large saucepan over medium heat and add the olive oil, bay leaves, Italian seasoning, and vegetable mixture. Sauté for 10 minutes, or until the water has evaporated.

3. Add the lentils, canned tomatoes, sun-dried tomatoes, tomato paste, capers, and stock. Stir to combine. Season to taste, reduce the heat to a gentle simmer, and cook uncovered for 25 minutes, to allow the liquid to evaporate, stirring occasionally. Remove the bay leaves.

4. Ten minutes before the sauce is ready (it should be thickening up and rich in flavor), cook the fettuccine al dente according to the package instructions (about 10 minutes).

5. Drain the pasta, transfer to serving plates, and stir in the sauce. Leave to sit for a few minutes, then grate some Parmesan or sprinkle nutritional yeast over it and serve.

Not ready to part with your meat? Meet me halfway—50 percent meat, 50 percent lentils—and you'll have a tasty meal that is responsible for almost 50 percent fewer greenhouse gas emissions.

Snacks

Whether you consider yourself a snacker or not, these recipes will get you thinking a little differently about these hunger satisfiers. Although snacks are notorious for neglecting the needs of our GM (low in fiber and high in added sugar and salt) and being problematic for those with food intolerances, it certainly doesn't have to be that way. In the pages to follow, you'll find plenty to inspire your savory snacking needs, each with a gut-health twist.

Sesame Kale Chips

You'll never look at kale the same way again. A game changer for all those who are anti-greens, it makes the perfect after-work snack or TV-time accompaniment.

1 teaspoon tahini
1 teaspoon garlic powder
1 tablespoon olive oil
Pinch of sea salt
5 cups (125 g) chopped kale
   leaves, destemmed
1 tablespoon sesame seeds

1. Preheat the oven to 350°F (180°C). Line two baking sheets with parchment paper.

2. Combine the tahini, garlic, oil, and salt in a large bowl. Add the kale and toss to evenly coat. Sprinkle with the sesame seeds.

3. Spread out the kale leaves on the prepared baking sheets, making sure not to crowd the pan. Bake for 10 minutes, or until crisp, then flip and cook for an additional 5 minutes. Keep a close eye on the chips and remove any that start to brown.

4. Allow to cool before digging in.

VARIATIONS

* For added flavor, add a teaspoon of an herb of your choice.
* Omit the garlic powder and replace the olive oil with garlic-infused olive oil to make this snack low-FODMAP.

Trio of Dips

In terms of nutrition, dips have been given a pretty bad rap. For many store-bought varieties, this may be warranted, but don't let that taint your perception of homemade dips. Their use goes way beyond dipping. I use them as spreads, dressings, sauces, fillings—and I add them to just about anything. They can transform any salad or veggie bowl, and they make a great afternoon snack when paired with veggie sticks or seeded crackers. Better still, these recipes are foolproof—add, blend, serve.

Classic Hummus

Butter's prebiotic sibling, providing nourishment not just for you but your GM, too.

One 15-ounce (425 g) can chickpeas, drained and rinsed (or 1½ cups/245 g cooked sprouted chickpeas; page 304)
1 garlic clove, crushed
¼ cup (60 ml) extra virgin olive oil
2 tablespoons fresh lemon juice
1 tablespoon tahini
½ teaspoon ground cumin
½ teaspoon smoked paprika, plus a pinch to serve (optional)
Pinch of salt
Fresh ground black pepper
Toasted pine nuts, to serve (optional)

1. Set aside 3 tablespoons of the chickpeas for serving.

2. Place the remaining chickpeas in a blender along with the garlic, oil, lemon juice, tahini, cumin, paprika, salt, pepper, and ¼ cup (60 ml) water and blend until completely smooth (for about 2 minutes). Taste as you go; you may like a little more lemon or salt.

3. Transfer to a serving dish and top with the reserved chickpeas and the pine nuts and/or paprika, if using.

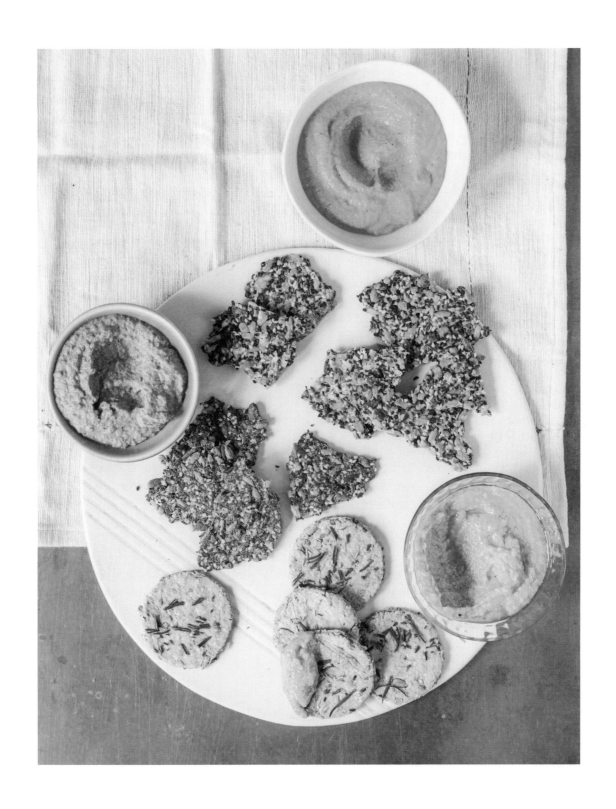

Pea and Mint Hummus

Creamy, minty—yum. This hummus is also garlic- and onion-free, which is a rare find in the world of dips. While the peas still do provide some FODMAPs (they are prebiotic, after all), you can include a half-portion for the FODMAP-lite approach. It could also be a good one to test when going through the reintroduction stage (see page 160).

2 cups (270 g) frozen peas, defrosted
2 tablespoons olive oil
2 teaspoons fresh lemon juice
1 teaspoon tahini
½ teaspoon ground cumin
Pinch of salt
1 handful fresh mint
Fresh ground black pepper
Mixed seeds, such as flaxseed, sunflower, pumpkin, and sesame, to serve

1. Blend the peas, oil, lemon juice, tahini, cumin, and salt with ¼ cup (60 ml) water in a blender until semi-smooth, about 1 minute.

2. Add the mint and season with pepper to taste. Blend for 1 minute, leaving a little of the texture from the mint leaves.

3. Serve topped with the seeds.

Harissa Dip

This vibrant dip, made with harissa, a hot pepper paste of Tunisian origin, is flavor-rich and nutrient-dense. Hazelnuts have been shown to help manage blood cholesterol, which is linked with lowering our risk of heart disease—flavor and health in one!

1⅓ cups (180 g) hazelnuts, toasted
One 12-ounce (340 g) jar of roasted peppers, drained
2 teaspoons fresh lemon juice
1 teaspoon honey, or sweetener of choice
1 teaspoon cumin seeds
1 teaspoon harissa
Pinch of salt
Twist of fresh ground black pepper

1. Set aside a few whole hazelnuts for serving.

2. Place the remaining ingredients in a blender and blend until a smooth paste forms (about 1 minute).

3. Serve topped with the reserved hazelnuts.

Trio of Crackers

Another one of my pantry staples. They're packed with plant-based protein and healthy fats—I doubt you'll find another cracker that lives up to these specs. I make a batch of each and enjoy them on rotation.

Seedy Oatcakes

Makes 12 oatcakes

I tend to keep a stash of these in my bag to keep me going in between meals on busy days. While the dough rests, consider some breathing (see page 184) or pelvic-floor (see page 196) exercises.

¾ cup (80 g) rolled oats
¼ cup (40 g) mixed seeds, such as flaxseed, sunflower, pumpkin, and sesame
Pinch of salt
1 tablespoon olive oil
¼ cup (60 ml) warm water
1 teaspoon dried rosemary (optional)

1. Preheat the oven to 375°F (190°C). Line a baking sheet with parchment paper.

2. Place the oats in a blender and pulse to form coarse crumbs.

3. Transfer to a large bowl. Add the seeds and salt, then mix in the oil and warm water. Mix with your hands to form a wet dough. Leave to rest somewhere warm for 10 minutes.

4. Place the dough in the middle of the prepared baking sheet. Place another sheet of parchment paper on top of the dough and, using a rolling pin or a glass bottle, spread the dough into a thin layer—the thinner, the better.

5. Remove the top sheet of paper and sprinkle the rosemary, if using, over the dough.

6. Using a cookie cutter (or a glass cup) roughly 2.5 inches (6 cm) in diameter, cut out oatcake circles, pressing firmly to cut through the seeds and removing any excess dough.

7. Bake for 20 to 25 minutes, or until golden brown.

VARIATION

* The rosemary can be replaced with basil and black pepper.

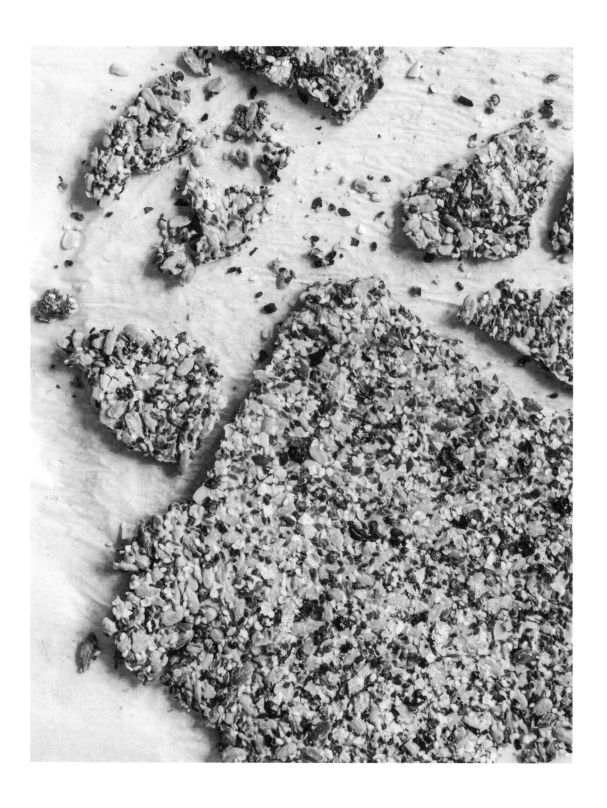

Cheesy Vegan Crackers

Gluten-free and dairy-free, but not flavor-free. Oh, and they're low-FODMAP, too.

1 cup (145 g) mixed seeds, such as flaxseed, sunflower, pumpkin, and sesame
¼ cup (35 g) buckwheat flour
¼ cup (25 g) ground flaxseeds
2½ tablespoons poppy seeds
2 tablespoons nutritional yeast
Pinch of salt
Twist of fresh ground black pepper
2 tablespoons olive oil
⅓ cup (80 ml) hot water
½ teaspoon dried thyme, to serve (optional)
Sea salt flakes, to serve (optional)

1. Preheat the oven to 350°F (180°C). Line a baking sheet with parchment paper.

2. In a large bowl, combine the mixed seeds, flour, ground flaxseeds, poppy seeds, nutritional yeast, salt, and pepper.

3. Slowly pour in the oil and hot water and, using your hands, make a wet dough. Leave to rest for 10 minutes somewhere warm.

4. Place the dough in the middle of the prepared baking sheet. Place another sheet of parchment paper on top of the dough and, using a rolling pin or a glass bottle, spread the dough into a thin layer—the thinner, the better.

5. Remove the top sheet of paper and sprinkle the thyme and salt flakes, if using, over the dough and gently press in.

6. Bake for 25 to 30 minutes, until slightly golden. Transfer to a cooling rack to cool completely, then break into cracker size of choice.

Spiced Chickpea and Sesame Seed Crackers

With a subtle hint of sesame seeds, this cracker is perfect for lifting any topping.

1 cup (145 g) mixed seeds, such as flaxseed, sunflower, and pumpkin
⅓ cup plus 2 tablespoons (50 g) chickpea flour
¼ cup (35 g) black (or white) sesame seeds
½ teaspoon cumin seeds
¼ teaspoon ground coriander
¼ teaspoon ground turmeric
Pinch of salt
Twist of fresh ground black pepper
2 tablespoons olive oil
⅓ cup (80 ml) hot water
½ teaspoon red pepper flakes (optional)
Sea salt flakes (optional)

1. Preheat the oven to 350°F (180°C). Line a baking sheet with parchment paper

2. In a large bowl, combine the mixed seeds, flour, sesame seeds, cumin, coriander, turmeric, salt, and pepper.

3. Slowly pour in the oil and hot water and, using your hands, make a wet dough. Leave to rest for 10 minutes somewhere warm.

4. Place the dough in the middle of the prepared baking sheet. Place another sheet of parchment paper on top of the dough and, using a rolling pin or a glass bottle, spread the dough into a thin layer—the thinner, the better.

5. Remove the top sheet of paper and sprinkle the red pepper flakes and sea salt flakes, if using, over the dough and gently press in.

6. Bake for 20 to 25 minutes, until slightly golden. Transfer to a cooling rack to cool completely, then break into cracker size of choice.

Sea Salt and Rosemary Legume Crunch

Our favorite bar snack—the flavor and crunch for me, and the prebiotics and polyphenols for my microbes. These tasty treats offer close to 5 grams of plant-based protein, making them a great topper on any Gut-Godness Bowl (page 246).

One 15-ounce (425 g) can mixed beans, or legume of choice, drained and rinsed
1 tablespoon olive oil
2 teaspoons dried rosemary
Pinch of salt

1. Preheat the oven to 400°F (200°C). Line a baking sheet with parchment paper.

2. Pat the beans dry, then toss in a bowl with the oil and seasonings.

3. Spread out on the prepared baking sheet. Bake for 15 to 20 minutes, until golden brown and crispy.

4. Allow to cool before digging in.

Spelt Wraps

It's near impossible to find an additive-free wrap on supermarket shelves (trust me, I've tried). So after playing around in the kitchen and discovering I could make them from scratch in less than five minutes, I've never looked back. I use this as my go-to base for the Mix-and-Match Sliders (page 234).

½ cup (65 g) whole-grain spelt flour
1 large egg
Pinch of salt
½ cup (120 ml) warm water
Oil, for cooking
1 teaspoon sesame seeds (optional)

1. Whisk together the flour, egg, salt, and warm water in a bowl for several minutes to form a thin, fluffy batter.

2. In a nonstick frying pan, warm a little oil over medium heat. Add ½ cup (120 ml) of the batter to the pan and swirl around the bottom so you get an even wrap. Sprinkle with sesame seeds, if using.

3. Cook for about 1 minute, until there are bubbles in the wrap and you can lift it to flip easily.

4. Cook on the other side for a minute, or until slightly brown. Wrap in a clean kitchen towel to keep the moisture in until ready to serve.

Spelt is a good source of prebiotics. For those following a strict low-FODMAP diet, fermented spelt (aka sourdough) is considered low-FODMAP, because microbes consume some of the FODMAPs.

Coconut-Crusted Green Beans with Zesty Yogurt Dip

Serves 4

The humble green bean, all dressed up. This one is a real crowd-pleaser, particularly among my foodie friends. The crispy, coconutty dippers are brought to life with the zesty yogurt dip, serving up a high-fiber, high-protein snack.

Coconut-Crusted Green Beans
Scant ½ cup (40 g) rolled oats
⅓ cup (25 g) unsweetened shredded coconut
2 teaspoons lime zest
½ teaspoon cumin seeds
½ teaspoon ground turmeric
½ teaspoon mustard seeds
Pinch of salt
Twist of fresh ground black pepper
½ teaspoon red pepper flakes (optional)
¾ cup (180 ml) milk of choice
¼ cup (30 g) coconut flour
14 ounces (400 g) green beans

Yogurt Dip
1 cup (240 g) Probiotic Yogurt (page 306)
¼ red onion, roughly sliced
1 teaspoon fresh lime juice
1 handful cilantro
Pinch of salt

1. Preheat the oven to 400°F (200°C). Line a baking sheet with parchment paper.

2. To make the green beans, use a blender to pulse the oats for a few seconds to form coarse crumbs.

3. Transfer to a large bowl and add the shredded coconut, lime zest, cumin, turmeric, mustard seeds, salt, pepper, and red pepper flakes, if using. Mix to combine.

4. Combine the milk and coconut flour in a second bowl. Leave to thicken for a few minutes.

5. Dip the beans into the milk and coconut flour batter (it will be quite thick, so use your hands to help coat) and then into the oat crumb mix. Place on the prepared baking sheet.

6. Bake for 20 minutes, or until golden and crispy.

7. While the beans are baking, place the dip ingredients in a blender and blend for a few seconds until roughly combined. Taste and adjust to preference. Serve with the crispy grean beans.

VARIATION

◆ For a low-FODMAP option, replace the onions with chives or the green part of scallions and opt for a lactose-free yogurt.

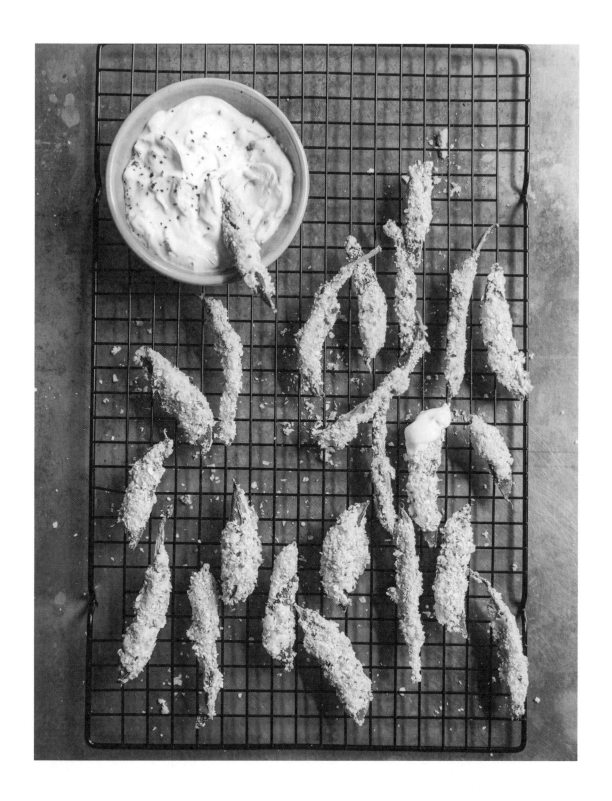

Sticky BBQ Vegan Wings

When your meat-loving brother asks for seconds, you know they must be good—finger-licking good. Unlike regular wings, these ones don't just feed you but are also a feast for your GM. You'll also be treated to 10 grams of plant-based protein per portion.

Vegan Wings
2 tablespoons self-rising flour
2 tablespoon soy milk
1 cauliflower, cut into bite-size florets
1 cup (100 g) almond meal
Scallions, to serve

BBQ Sauce
⅔ cup (170 g) ketchup
2 teaspoons soy sauce
2 teaspoons vegan Worcestershire sauce
1 teaspoon smoked paprika
1 teaspoon chipotle flakes
½ teaspoon garlic powder

1. Preheat the oven to 375°F (190°C). Line a baking sheet with parchment paper.

2. To make the wings, combine the flour and milk in a small bowl to form a thin batter.

3. Dry the cauliflower florets, then dunk them in the batter. Shake off any excess batter, then coat with the almond meal.

4. Place on the prepared baking sheet and bake for 20 minutes, turning once halfway through.

5. To make the sauce, combine all the ingredients in a small saucepan and simmer for 2 minutes.

4. Remove the cauliflower from the oven and dip each floret into the sauce in the saucepan. Return to the baking sheet.

5. Bake for an additional 5 to 10 minutes, until the "wings" are crispy and the sauce has caramelized. Sprinkle with scallions and serve.

Plant chemicals found in cauliflower have been shown to directly support the health of the immune cells that line our intestine, at least in animal studies.[8]

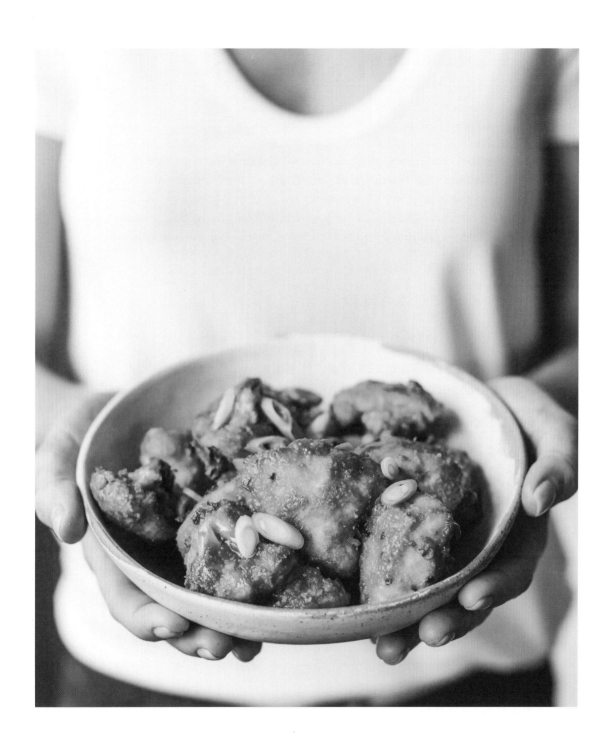

Desserts

Sweet treats can be a real mood-booster. But imagine ones that don't lift just your mood but the mood of your GM, too. Well, imagine no more, because this is what my sweet snacks are all about! Whether you're looking for that 3:00 PM pick-me-up, a movie-night treat, or a snack to pull out when you're looking to turn some heads, I've got you covered.

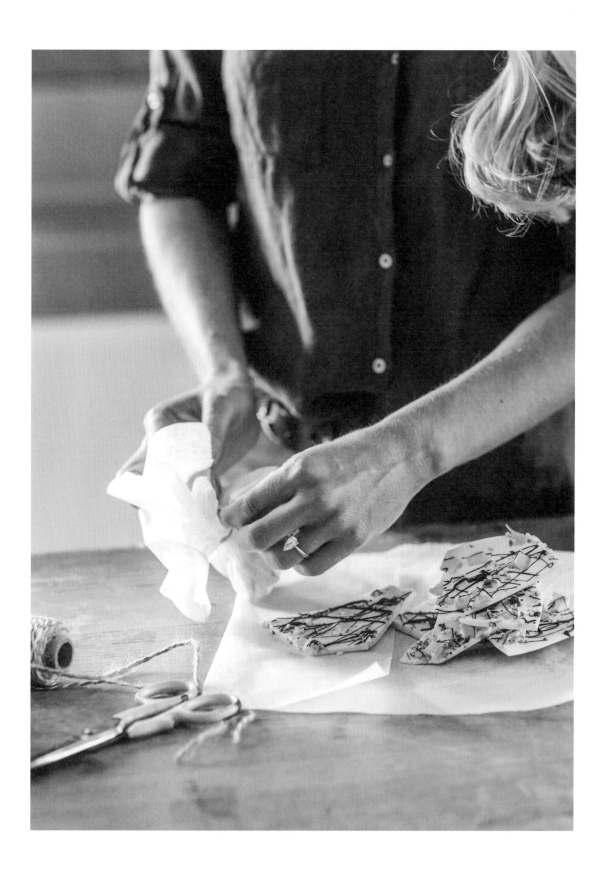

Raw Carrot Cake Balls

Makes twelve 1-ounce (25 g) balls

An indulgent treat that's also high in fiber and loaded with polyphenols—yes, it's possible! A single batch is never enough. Freeze in single portions and enjoy as a pre-gym snack or a midmorning boost.

4 Medjool dates, pitted (about 2 ounces/60 g)
½ cup (50 g) almond meal
¼ cup (25 g) rolled oats
1 large carrot, grated (about 3.5 ounces/100 g)
¼ cup (15 g) coconut flakes
2 tablespoons ground flaxseed
1 teaspoon ground allspice
½ teaspoon ground cinnamon
½ teaspoon ground ginger
1 teaspoon grated fresh ginger, if you like extra zing! (optional)
1 teaspoon vanilla extract
¼ cup (25 g) walnuts

Coating (choose 1; optional)
Unsweetened shredded coconut
Poppy seeds
Whole or ground flaxseeds
Crushed nuts
Melted dark chocolate

1. Place the dates, almond meal, and oats in a food processor and blend until everything is roughly combined.

2. Add the carrot, coconut flakes, flaxseed, allspice, cinnamon, ground ginger, fresh ginger, if using, and the vanilla and blend again. The mixture should be moist but not so wet that you can't roll it (if it's too wet, add an extra sprinkle of oats).

3. Using a walnut half as the center, form a ball around it with the mixture. Leave naked or roll in your coating of choice. Transfer to a large plate or baking sheet. Repeat until all the dough has been used up.

4. Transfer the balls to the fridge to firm up for at least 2 hours before eating.

A handful of walnuts a day for 3 weeks has been shown to increase microbes that produce the beneficial short-chain fatty acid butyrate.[9] The walnuts also decreased specific compounds that are linked with colon cancer.

Fudgy Black Bean Brownies

I serve this tasty treat to all the fussy eaters in my life. Loaded with polyphenols and prebiotics, their microbes love me for it. You'll need cupcake liners for this recipe.

¾ cup (80 g) rolled oats
½ cup (125 g) drained and rinsed canned black beans
1 large extra-ripe banana, peeled (about 4 ounces/120 g)
8 small prunes, pitted (about 1.5 ounces/40 g)
6 Medjool dates, pitted (about 3 ounces/90 g)
2 large eggs
¼ cup (20 g) cocoa powder
1 teaspoon baking powder
Pinch of salt
½ cup (120 ml) milk of choice
1 teaspoon vanilla extract
¼ cup (50 g) dark chocolate chips
¼ cup (30 g) chopped walnuts or 2 tablespoons crunchy peanut butter (optional)

Toppings
Probiotic Yogurt (page 306)
Honey (optional)
Frozen berries

1. Preheat the oven to 400°F (200°C). Line a muffin pan with cupcake liners.

2. Place the oats, beans, banana, eggs, prunes, dates, cocoa powder, baking powder, salt, milk, and vanilla in a blender and blend until completely smooth (around 3 minutes).

3. Spoon the mixture into the prepared muffin cups. Dot in the chocolate chips and nuts, if using.

4. Bake for 10 to 12 minutes, until a knife comes out clean when inserted in the center of a muffin, then allow to cool in the pan for 5 minutes.

5. Before serving, top with a dollop of yogurt (sweetened with honey, if using) and frozen berries of choice.

6. To store the brownies, wrap each portion individually and freeze. Next time you're craving a sweet snack, warm in the microwave before topping and digging in.

There is a convincing body of evidence to support the role of the polyphenols found in cocoa (flavanols) in lowering blood pressure, and also in improving clarity of thought as we age.[10] Another study has shown that a single dose of a flavanol-rich chocolate drink counteracted the effects of sleep deprivation on memory in healthy women[11]—sign me up!

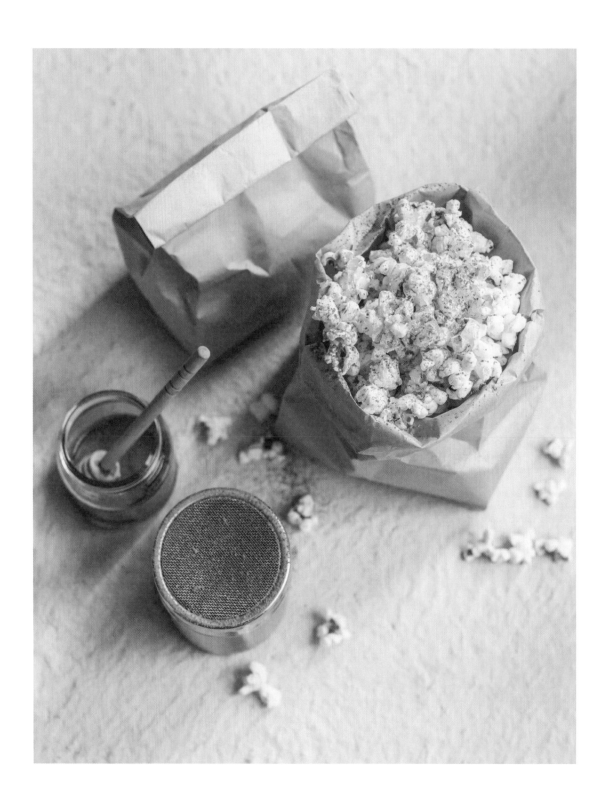

Cinnamon-Spiced Microwave Popcorn

When it comes to those afternoon sweet cravings, this high-fiber snack certainly hits the spot. Quick, easy, and oh so tasty. You'll need a brown paper bag for this recipe.

¼ cup (50 g) popcorn kernels
1 teaspoon honey
¼ teaspoon ground cinnamon

1. Pour the corn kernels into a brown paper bag and fold the top over twice to seal.

2. Microwave on high for about 3 minutes, or until you hear a pause of about 3 seconds between pops.

3. Leave to stand for 20 seconds, then carefully open the bag.

4. Drizzle in the honey, followed by the cinnamon. Refold the top of the bag and shake to combine.

VARIATIONS

- Experiment with other flavor combinations, such as olive oil (2 teaspoons), curry powder (½ teaspoon), and ground coriander (½ teaspoon), or vinegar (1 teaspoon) and salt (½ teaspoon).

- If you don't have a microwave, don't let that get between you and your hopes of cinnamon-spiced popcorn. Pour in a small amount of oil to coat the bottom of the biggest saucepan you have, covered with a glass lid. Set it over medium heat and add in a single layer of kernels before covering with the lid. As soon as you see the popcorn beginning to pop, continuously shake the pan gently over the burner to ensure the kernels don't burn. After a minute or so, once the popping has slowed down significantly, remove from the heat. Allow it to cool briefly, then drizzle on the honey and cinnamon. Transfer to a bowl and dig in.

Lemon Curd Tartlets with a Chia and Cashew Crust

A gut-boosting twist on my favorite dessert—you'll find live microbes in the curd and prebiotics in the crust. Beware: Your GM may not let you stop at just one.

Chia and Cashew Crust
½ cup (65 g) cashews
2½ tablespoons chia seeds
⅓ cup (25 g) unsweetened shredded coconut
⅓ cup plus 1 tablespoon (40 g) rolled oats
4 Medjool dates, pitted and chopped (about 2 ounces/60 g)
Oil, for greasing

Lemon Curd Filling
1 teaspoon lemon zest, plus extra for garnish
¼ cup plus 2 teaspoons (70 ml) fresh lemon juice (from about 2 lemons), plus more as needed
3 tablespoons honey, or sweetener of choice
1 tablespoon arrowroot starch
⅔ cup plus 2 teaspoons (170 g) Probiotic Yogurt (page 306)

1. Preheat the oven to 325°F (165°C).

2. To make the crust, place all the ingredients in a blender with ¼ cup (60 ml) water and blend until roughly combined. With your hands, roll the mix together to form a sticky dough and allow to rest for 10 minutes in the fridge.

3. While the dough is resting, grease a mini muffin pan with your oil of choice.

4. Once the dough has firmed up, press a tablespoonful into each mold. Use your fingertip to evenly spread the dough across the base and sides.

5. Bake for 15 minutes, or until golden brown. Set aside to cool.

6. Meanwhile, to make the lemon curd filling, combine the lemon zest, lemon juice, honey, and arrowroot in a small saucepan over low heat. Stir vigorously with a wooden spatula until the mix becomes a thick gel.

7. Remove from the heat and let cool for 1 to 2 minutes, then stir in the yogurt. Taste as you go, and adjust the lemon to taste.

8. Allow the tartlet crusts to cool completely before dolloping the curd into each one. Refrigerate for at least 4 hours to set. Garnish with extra lemon zest.

VARIATIONS

◆ Prefer a crunchy tartlet crust? Make the lemon curd first and allow to set, covered, in the fridge for 4 hours. Bake the crusts and allow to cool. When ready to serve, dollop the thick curd into each crust.

◆ For a nut-free option, omit the cashews, up the oats to ¾ cup (80 g), and add one extra date.

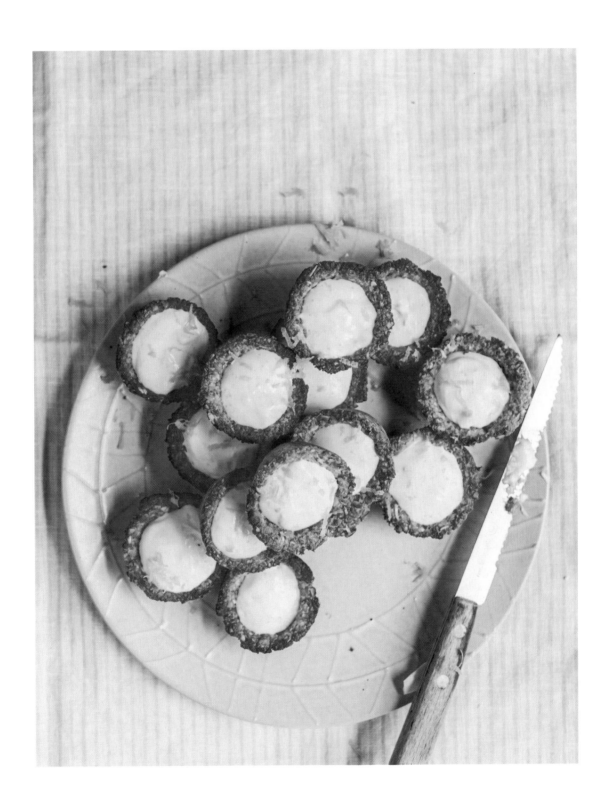

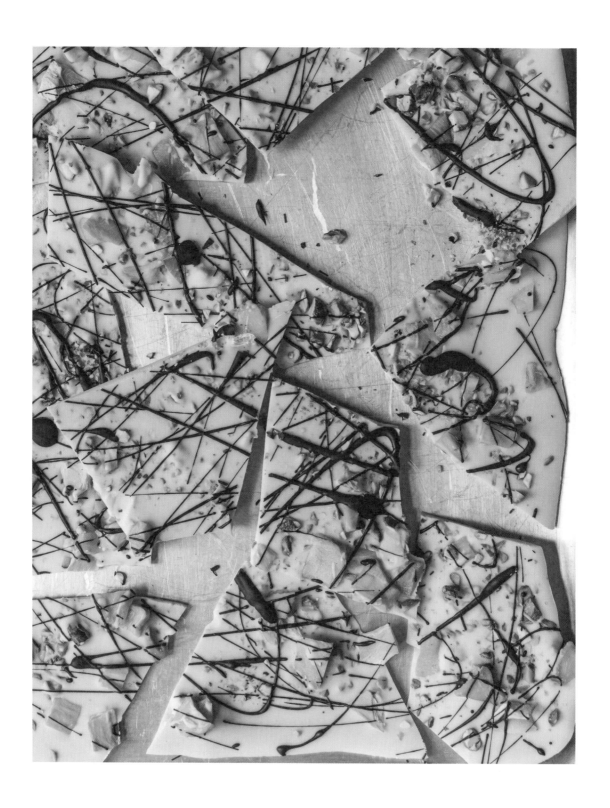

Prebiotic Chocolate Bark

I always make these for my friends and family at Easter, wrapped up in tissue paper and tied with craft string—I'd hate for everyone's microbes to feel left out of the celebrations.

7 ounces (200 g) good-quality white chocolate

2 teaspoons extra virgin olive oil

½ cup (50 g) dried mango, diced

½ cup (50 g) crushed pistachios

2 ounces (50 g) good-quality dark chocolate (70 percent or more cocoa solids)

1. Place the white chocolate in a small microwave-safe bowl and microwave for 40 to 60 seconds, stirring vigorously every 15 seconds, until melted.

2. Add the oil to the melted white chocolate, followed by half the dried mango and pistachios, and stir to combine. Pour the mixture onto a lined baking sheet, thinly spreading it out. Dot in the rest of the mango and pistachios. Place in the fridge for 5 minutes to set.

3. Meanwhile, in a separate bowl, melt the dark chocolate in the microwave, as in step 1.

4. Once the white chocolate is firm, use a fork to drizzle on the dark chocolate with whipping movements. Chill in the fridge for 30 minutes or until rock solid, then remove and break the bark into pieces.

The darker the chocolate, the higher the percentage of cocoa, which means the more polyphenols. This may explain why dark chocolate has been linked with decreased risk of heart disease and diabetes ... albeit in moderation. In fact, several studies have found that daily consumption of cocoa significantly lowered participants' blood pressure—a key risk factor for heart disease.[12]

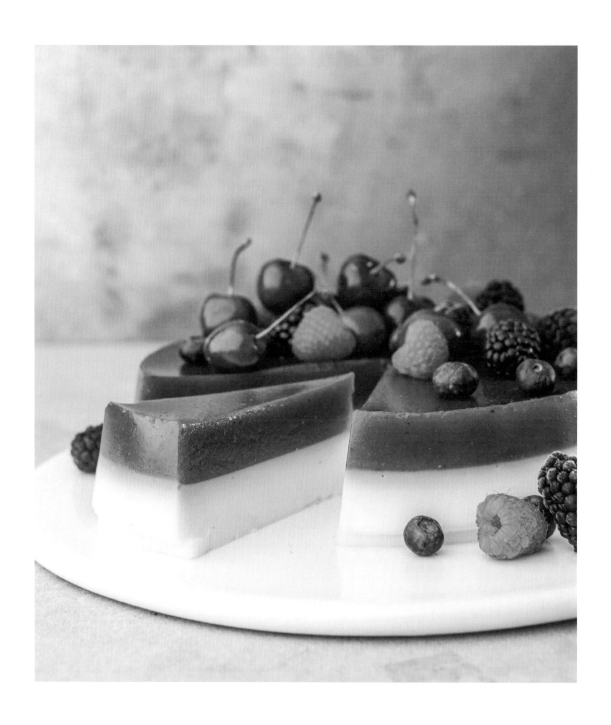

Live Berry and Coconut Jelly

I've never met a jelly I didn't like, but this takes things to the next level. It's also won the heart of my two-year-old nephew = a proud Aunty moment!

Coconut Jelly
5 gelatin sheets (see Notes)
½ cup (120 ml) warm water
1 cup (240 g) plain probiotic coconut yogurt
2 tablespoons honey, or sweetener of choice
Neutral oil or oil spray, for greasing

Berry Jelly
5 gelatin sheets (see Notes)
1 cup (240 ml) warm water
1 cup (140 g) frozen berries or mango
2 tablespoons honey, or sweetener of choice

1. To make the coconut jelly, place the gelatin sheets in a bowl and cover with cold water for 5 minutes to allow the gelatin to soften, then drain off the water. Add the warm water and stir until the gelatin has dissolved, then allow to cool.

2. Meanwhile, lightly grease a gelatin mold or 6-inch (15 cm) round cake pan. Combine the coconut yogurt and honey in a bowl before slowly stirring in the gelatin. Mix until smooth.

3. Pour into the bottom of the mold, leaving room for the berry jelly (see Notes). Place in the fridge to set overnight (or for at least 4 hours) before preparing the berry jelly.

4. To make the berry jelly, place the gelatin sheets in a bowl and cover with cold water for 5 minutes, then drain off the water.

5. Place the berries and warm water in a small blender and allow to defrost for a few minutes. Blend for a few seconds to form a rough purée. Transfer to a saucepan and simmer over low heat for 5 minutes, stirring every minute or so. Remove from the heat.

6. Place a metal sieve on top of a bowl and pour the purée through it. With the back of a spoon, push all the pulp through the sieve, leaving just the seeds. Don't throw out the seeds! They make a great addition to your breakfast granola.

7. Add the softened gelatin to the purée and stir until dissolved. Cool to room temperature, then spoon on top of the set coconut jelly. Pop back in the fridge for 6 to 8 hours to set.

NOTES:

♦ *Want a bit of extra texture? Stir ⅔ cup (50 g) unsweetened shredded coconut into the coconut layer before leaving to set.*

♦ *If you can't find gelatin sheets, use 1½ packets (or 1 tablespoon + ½ teaspoon Knox gelatin powder for each jelly. Sprinkle the powder into ¼ cup (60 ml) cold water and let stand 5 minutes. Then, for the coconut jelly, add only ¼ cup warm water and stir, as you would with the gelatin sheets, and for the berry jelly, use only ¾ cup (180 ml) warm water.*

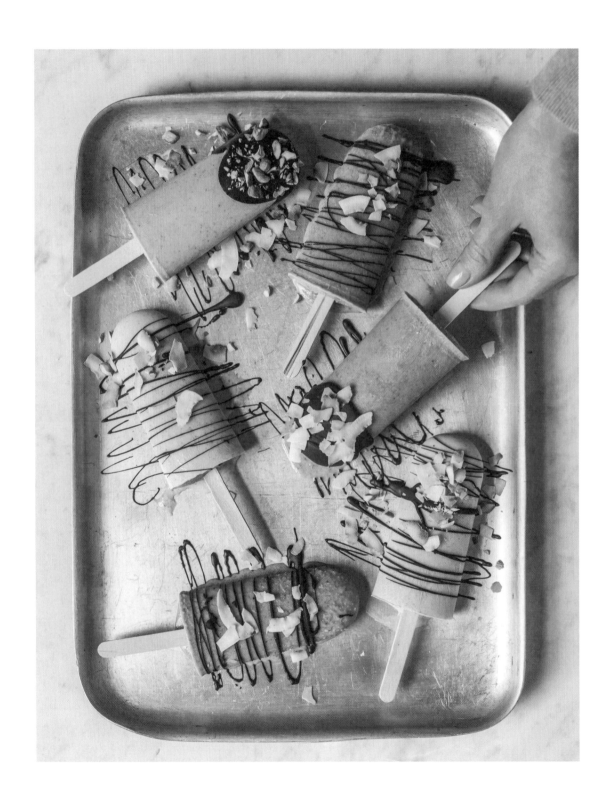

Synbiotic Ice Pops

When convenience and taste align, you know you're onto a winner. No need for a fancy ice cream machine—this combo draws on the creaminess of bananas and the richness of thick probiotic yogurt to deliver gut goodness on a stick.

Ice Cream
1 extra ripe banana, peeled (about 3.5 ounces/100 g)
2 Medjool dates, chopped and stirred into a paste with 1 tablespoon boiling water
1 cup (240 g) plain probiotic full-fat yogurt (coconut or dairy, such as Probiotic Yogurt, page 306)
1 teaspoon vanilla extract

Flavors (choose one)

NUTTY PISTACHIO
(Serves 6)
½ cup (50 g) shelled pistachios
10 baby spinach leaves

RAW BANOFFEE
(Serves 8)
1 ripe banana, peeled (about 3.5 ounces/100 g)
½ cup (120 g) coconut yogurt
⅓ cup (70 g) almond butter

Extras (optional)
Dark chocolate
Coconut flakes

1. To make the ice cream, place all of the ingredients in a blender and blend until smooth.

2. Add your chosen flavor ingredients to the ice cream mixture. Roughly blend to your desired texture.

3. Spoon into popsicle molds, insert sticks or handles, and place in the freezer for at least 4 hours.

4. Once the ice pops have set, if desired, warm the dark chocolate in the microwave for 40 to 60 seconds, stirring vigorously every 15 seconds until melted.

5. Remove the ice pops from the molds (if you struggle to get them out, dip the outside of the mold in warm water for a few seconds). Lay them on a baking sheet (lined for easy cleanup), drizzle with the chocolate, and sprinkle with coconut flakes, if using.

VARIATIONS

* Keep things simple and just mix in 2 ounces (55 g) of your fruit of choice to the ice cream.

* Want to up the presentation stakes? Layer the molds with different flavors, freezing before adding each one.

Can bacteria survive the freeze? You bet. According to research in the Journal of Dairy Science, *they can't handle the heat, but they can handle the cold.*[13]

Substituting the cream with yogurt will save you 86 percent in greenhouse gas emissions.[14]

Welcome to Fermenting!

What Is Fermentation?

Fermentation describes the process by which bacteria and yeast predigest, or transform, food and drinks. In doing so, they produce a range of by-products, such as vitamins, beneficial organic acids and other bioactive compounds, flavor compounds, gases, and, in some cases, alcohol.

Unlike many fermenting advocates, who were born and raised on fermented goodness, fermenting isn't "in my blood." In fact, if you'd asked me only five years ago, I probably would have told you it was a bit too hippie-dippie for me. But now, I've realized I couldn't have been more wrong.

What began as a work experiment aimed at boosting my gut microbes rapidly turned into a deep-seated passion that's now embedded into my daily routine. During the experiment, in which I began to eat fermented foods every day—alternating between kimchi, kefir, kombucha, and sauerkraut—I noticed several things: I felt mentally and physically better than ever (anecdotal evidence alert: yes, that's the lowest-quality "evidence" there is); my weekly grocery bill had gotten smaller (hello, new shoes); and, above all, the thing that really got me hooked—the flavors. The microbes involved in fermentation possess the most extraordinary "culinary" skills. Think about the most flavorful foods out there—aged cheeses, olives, chocolate, vanilla, coffee, wine, and soy sauce, among others. None of these would be possible without microbes.

Before we get into the science of it, I want to tackle a few of the rumors about fermenting that could deter any budding fermenters out there.

RUMOR 1: Fermenting Is Labor-Intensive

Fermenting reminds me of a slow cooker: It takes surprisingly little effort—once you've prepared it, you just leave it, allow the microbes to do the heavy lifting, and carry on with your activities. You later return to a dish that's transformed and ready to serve. It's true that some fermented foods can be a labor of love, but, for those who are busy, there are plenty of time-efficient options. Kefir, yogurt, and sourdough wraps all take about two minutes to prepare. You leave them overnight, and, by morning, they're ready to enjoy. Other ferments, such as kimchi and sauerkraut, take a little longer to prepare, but every few months I spend an afternoon making them in bulk—and it's so worth it.

RUMOR 2: **Fermenting Is Dangerous**

Growing up in a generation where total sterilization was gospel and every household surface was soaked in antibacterial products, I was naturally a little intimidated by the perceived risk attached to fermenting. But it turns out the risk of food poisoning is far greater when you eat out at a restaurant. In fact, it's been suggested that regular consumption of traditional fermented foods may protect you from gut infections such as food poisoning—although I must admit most of the research is from test-tube studies.[15]

You do need to keep your wits about you, use your senses (yes, the good old sniff test will tell you if something is rancid), and, if in doubt, ask for help (there is a very active Facebook fermenting community that is free to join).

RUMOR 3: **Fermenting Is Not Suitable for Kids**

It's actually just the opposite, and, in fact, I can't think of a better way to engage kids in science, food, and healthy eating. Microbes, particularly yeast, do produce alcohol, but the alcohol levels in most types of ferments are below detection levels (i.e., considered alcohol-free), thanks to bacteria that convert the alcohol into beneficial organic acids.

> As with dietary fiber, going from little to loads of fermented food within a few days can, in some people, trigger gut symptoms, such as extra gas and bloating—it's like a microbial party in a normally quiet neighborhood. It's best to gradually increase the amount in your diet over several weeks. People with histamine sensitivity (see page 122) may need to limit their intake. And those with a weakened immune system or who are pregnant should discuss with a healthcare professional first.

The Process

Despite there being hundreds of different types of ferments, there are three main principles that underpin them all.

- **MICROBES:** No surprises here: To ferment, you need live microbes. There are two main types of ferments, determined by where the microbes come from. "Wild ferments," like kimchi, use the microbes naturally found on plants and in the air, whereas "culture-based ferments," like yogurt, involve adding a select group of microbes.

- **FOOD FOR THE MICROBES:** The second most important ingredient is the food to keep the microbes alive. Without this, the microbes will become too weak to ferment. Like us, different microbes prefer different foods, which is why you need to be selective about the type of foods you feed different microbes. For example, the microbes used to make traditional yogurt eat lactose (milk sugar), which is found in milk from animals. If you try adding these microbes to a lactose-free milk (e.g., plant-based milk), they starve, and you are left with a watery mess instead of a thick, creamy yogurt.

- **SELECTIVE ENVIRONMENT:** Just like some people prefer cold weather and others hot, different microbes prefer different environments. Ensuring the environment matches the microbes you're trying to grow will make sure you cultivate the right ones. For example, when fermenting vegetables, you need to create a salty, oxygen-free environment to support the growth of the lactic-acid bacteria while preventing the growth of fungi (surface mold) that can spoil your ferment. When it comes to the temperature, although most ferments do have an ideal temperature (detailed in each recipe), I've found most ferments can be pretty flexible. Also, within your home, there are microclimates that you can make use of across seasons. For example, in the winter, I move my ferments closer to the radiator. As a rule of thumb, microbes get rather sleepy and less active in cooler temperatures (which means ferments take longer) and more energized and active in warmer climates (ferments take less time).

Sprouting

One of the things I miss most about home is my mom's vegetable patch. There is something therapeutic about the process: planting the seeds, watching out for the first sprout, the daily watering, and, finally, harvesting, preparing, and eating the vegetables. While I certainly don't have the space (or time) to recreate my mom's luscious garden, I've found much of this gratification with sprouting.

The thing about sprouting is that anybody can do it anywhere; you don't need any fancy equipment or a lot of time. Sprouts are a great source of fiber and micronutrients and contain an array of polyphenols and other beneficial bioactive compounds. Studies have also shown that some types of sprouts contain manifold more bioactive compounds with anticancer benefits (albeit in test-tube studies[16]), compared to the fully grown plants. Like fermenting, sprouting also decreases some types of antinutrients and activates certain enzymes, therefore increasing the availability of several nutrients, such as amino acids (protein building blocks), and minerals, such as iron, calcium, magnesium, and zinc.

That's not to say we should be ditching the fully grown plants and replacing them with sprouts; I consider them more of an extra kick of nutrients than the bulk of my diet. For those wondering if there are any studies in humans, there aren't many. One trial did find that 2 ounces (60 grams) of lentil sprouts eaten daily over eight weeks improved cholesterol levels as well as blood sugar control in overweight people with type 2 diabetes.[17] Sounds impressive, right? But annoyingly, because they didn't compare this to unsprouted lentils, it's impossible to know whether it was the act of sprouting or just the lentils themselves.

Rest assured: It's not just about the health benefits—the nutty flavor and crunchy texture of sprouts also make them a crowd-pleaser. Toss them into a salad, stir-fry, curry, burger, or omelet. While just about any bean, grain, vegetable, nut, or seed can be sprouted, some are easier (and safer) than others. If you're new to sprouting, I recommend starting with an easy win—alfalfa seeds (see page 304).

Raw Slaw

Move over coleslaw, there's a new slaw in town—meet raw slaw (aka sauerkraut): It's where the flavors (and microbes) are. I put this on top of my burgers and eat it as a side to BBQ dishes. The process is simple—slice, salt, squash, submerge . . . sit.

10 ounces (300 g) Napa cabbage (about ½ small head), or cabbage of choice (I like to combine red and white varieties)

¾ teaspoon (4 g) sea salt (or any non-iodized salt free of anticaking agents)

1 teaspoon white miso paste

1 scallion, roughly chopped

1 teaspoon grated ginger

Equipment

One 16-ounce (or 500 ml) airtight jar with lid, sterilized

Glass weight or small glass jar, to keep the ferment submerged

1. Rinse each of the cabbage leaves under running water (to get rid of any residual soil) before chopping to your desired thickness.

2. Put the sliced cabbage into a large bowl, then add the salt. Wash your hands, then firmly massage in the salt until the cabbage is bruised—this process helps the microbes get into the cabbage cell walls, where they will do their thing.

3. Pour a tablespoon of the cabbage juice into a small mug and stir in the miso paste. Pour the mixture over the cabbage, then add the scallion and ginger and continue massaging the cabbage until it is limp and everything is combined.

4. Transfer to the jar and, using your fist, punch down the slaw, pushing out all the air bubbles so that the mixture is completely submerged and there is a layer of juice separating the slaw and the air above it.

5. To keep it submerged, place a glass weight or mini jar on top of the slaw.

6. Screw the lid onto the jar and leave at room temperature (ideally, 65 to 70°F/18 to 22°C), out of direct sunlight. Each day, check on your ferment and release any gas that has built up by unscrewing the lid a little to let it escape.

7. After 7 days (more in colder climates, fewer in warmer climates), your slaw is ready to taste. If you're new to fermenting, that might be sufficient time; if you prefer a stronger acidic flavor, continue to ferment for up to 4 weeks, testing weekly. Once it has reached your preferred flavor, pop it into the fridge for a few days to stop the fermentation (this puts the microbes to sleep), then dig in.

The Importance of Salt

I am normally all for limiting salt in our diets, but when it comes to fermented vegetables, salt has several important functions. 1) It creates a selective environment that supports the beneficial lactic acid bacteria, which, unlike many microbes, are rather salt-tolerant. 2) Through a process known as osmosis, salt helps to draw the juices out of the vegetables, providing the liquid needed to submerge them. 3) It preserves the crisp crunch of cabbage that would otherwise turn mushy.

The salt "sweet spot" is around 1.5 to 2 percent by weight of the vegetables. It's best to weigh your salt because, depending on the grain size, volumes can yield very different weights. If you're limiting your salt, ferments can still work with lower levels of salt, but they won't last as long. Non-iodized salt free of anticaking agents is best.

For those worried about the effect of added salt on blood pressure, there is some evidence to suggest it's probably not as detrimental as salt from processed foods because of the potassium found in vegetables.[18] Potassium-rich vegetables are known to lower blood pressure and therefore may offset the impact of the salt. One study reported that a daily intake of 7.5 ounces (210 grams) of kimchi for seven days did not affect blood pressure, although this was in people with healthy blood pressure.[19] Nonetheless, if you do have high blood pressure or are concerned, it's a good idea to discuss with your healthcare professional. You might also like to do a mini trial on yourself, testing the impact of regularly consuming fermented vegetables on your blood pressure over a few weeks.

Tap Water

Chlorine is another microbe inhibitor, which is why it's often added to drinking water. Rather than buying filtered or spring water, you can dechlorinate your tap water by boiling it in an uncovered pot, so that the chlorine can escape. Allow it to cool before using (hot water will kill the microbes).

Mold

If you notice any surface mold growing, it may be because you didn't completely submerge your vegetables. While some people say you can just scrape it off and continue fermenting, I like to play it safe, which means ditching it and starting again.

Kimchi

An iconic condiment in Korean culture, this ancient flavor bomb is said to be one of the secrets behind Koreans' long and healthy lives. In fact, a study published in the *Lancet* has forecasted that South Korean women will be the first in the world to have an average life expectancy above ninety years by 2030.[20] Kimchi is spicy, tangy, and delicious. Enjoy with eggs (my favorite), salads, or feta on crackers—the options are endless.

7 ounces (200 g) Napa cabbage (about ⅓ small head), or cabbage of choice

1½ tablespoons (25 g) sea salt (don't worry, you won't be eating this!)

2 cups (500 ml) filtered or dechlorinated water

1 carrot, grated

½ cup (50 g) julienned daikon radish

1 scallion, sliced

1 garlic clove, thinly sliced

1 teaspoon grated ginger

1 teaspoon gochugaru (see Note)

1 tablespoon tamari or soy sauce

Equipment

One 16-ounce (or 500 ml) glass jar with lid, sterilized

Glass weight or small glass jar, to keep the ferment submerged

1. Rinse the cabbage leaves under running water (to get rid of any residual soil) before chopping to your desired thickness.

2. Put the cabbage and salt in a bowl. Firmly massage the salt into the cabbage.

3. Pour the water over the cabbage and submerge it by sitting a plate on top. Let it soak for 2 hours.

4. Drain and rinse three times to get rid of the excess salt. Squeeze out any excess water and return the cabbage to the bowl.

5. Add the carrot, daikon, scallion, garlic, ginger, gochugaru, and tamari and mix well, then transfer to the jar and, using your fist, punch down so that the mixture is submerged and there's a layer of juice separating the raw kimchi and the air above.

6. To keep it submerged, place a glass weight or mini jar on top of the kimchi.

7. Screw the lid on and leave at room temperature (ideally, 65 to 70°F/18 to 22°C), out of direct sunlight. Each day, check on your kimchi and release any gas that has built up by unscrewing the lid a little to let it escape.

8. After 3 days (more in colder climates, less in warmer climates) your kimchi is ready for its first taste. If you're missing that acidic bite, leave it for an extra day or two.

9. Once it's reached your preferred flavor, pop it in the fridge with the lid sealed tight to trap in the gas (this will create the fizziness of traditional kimchi). Leave it for 2 weeks to allow the flavors to develop.

NOTE: *Gochugaru, Korean red pepper flakes, is available online or at Asian grocers. If you can't find it, use ½ teaspoon cayenne and ½ teaspoon paprika.*

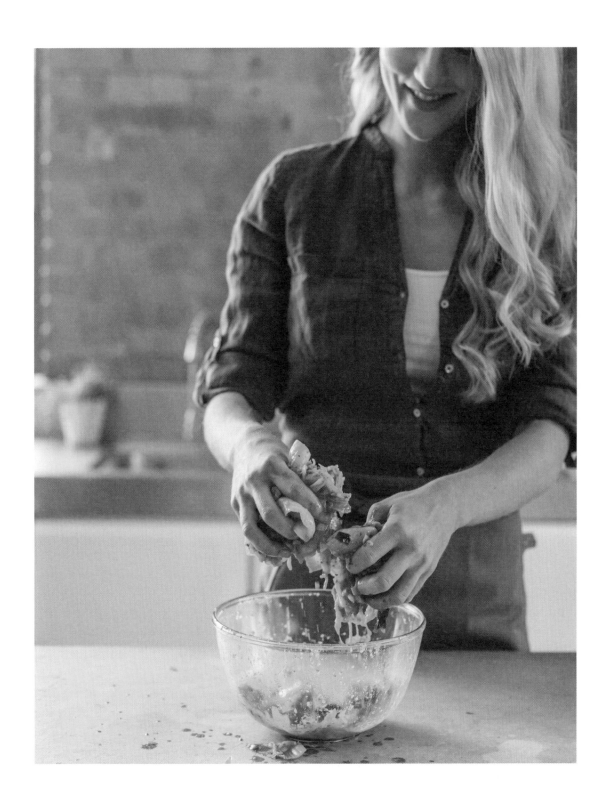

Sourdough Starter

When I first started making sourdough, I was gifted a starter from my local artisan bakery. As I became more confident with the process, I wanted to challenge myself to see whether I could make a starter from scratch. It does take more time and requires a bit more fermenting experience, but it's something you only need to do once—if you look after it, it will keep forever.

Each day for 7 days
¼ cup bread flour
¼ cup (60 ml) lukewarm filtered or dechlorinated water

Equipment
One 16-ounce (or 400 ml) glass jar
Cheesecloth (to cover)
Rubber band

1. Day 1: Place the flour in the glass jar, then stir in the water gradually, to prevent clumping. Cover with the cheesecloth and secure with a rubber band. Leave overnight at room temperature (ideally, 68 to 75°F/20 to 24°C).

2. Day 2: In the morning, stir and cover again. That evening, stir before discarding all but 1 tablespoon of your floury mix, now known as the "starter." Add fresh flour and water, repeating step 1.

3. Days 3 to 7: Repeat step 2.

4. Day 8: In the morning, stir. Your starter should appear fluffy, with a network of bubbles throughout, and have a slightly sour, yeasty smell. This means it's ready to be used in your sourdough recipes. If there are only a few bubbles, continue feeding your starter for a few more days until it becomes more active.

Why throw out most of your starter? I am anti food waste, but this step is important when making a starter. This is because overwhelming the starter each day with more fresh food than there is starter lowers the acidity and gives the yeast a competitive advantage.

STORAGE TIP: *Store your starter in the fridge, sealed with an airtight lid. As you use your starter, replace with equal parts flour and water to ensure you maintain it—you don't want to have to start again from scratch. At a minimum, feed your starter once a week with 1 tablespoon flour and 1 tablespoon water. Mix well and leave on the kitchen counter, covered with the cheesecloth, for 1 to 2 hours before returning to the fridge with the lid secured.*

Sourdough Wraps

I love sourdough bread, but the hours of leavening and dough stretching mean I rarely get time to make it. Instead of settling for the store-bought stuff, I decided to experiment with fermented wraps. A few attempts later, a time-efficient sourdough victory was mine! It's now become my go-to sourdough fix.

⅔ cup (100 g) whole wheat flour
½ cup plus 2 tablespoons (150 ml) filtered or dechlorinated water
1 teaspoon active sourdough starter (page 299)
Pinch of salt
Oil, for frying

1. In a glass or ceramic bowl, whisk the flour, the water, and the sourdough starter together. Cover with a clean cloth secured with a rubber band and leave at room temperature (ideally, 68 to 75°F/20 to 24°C), out of direct sunlight, for 6 to 8 hours (plus or minus a few hours, depending on the temperature), or until the batter becomes fluffy, with a network of bubbles throughout. If you prefer a sourer wrap, leave for longer. When ready for cooking, stir in the salt.

2. Warm a little oil in a nonstick frying pan over medium heat. Add ½ cup (120 ml) of the batter to the pan and swirl around to form an even layer.

3. Cook for about 1 minute, until there are bubbles in the wrap and you can lift it to flip easily.

4. Cook on the other side for 1 minute or until slightly brown. Wrap in a clean kitchen towel to keep in the moisture until ready to serve. Best eaten warm.

What's the deal with sourdough and fermented bread? The delicious taste and chewiness aside, sourdough fermentation has been shown to lower the blood sugar response to bread and also to increase the bioavailability of nutrients (meaning that more nutrients are freed up for absorption). Better still, the microbes found in sourdough starter have been shown to produce bioactive compounds with impressive antioxidant activity. Winning on all fronts.

Dairy Kefir

Kefir, a cousin to yogurt, has the same creaminess but provides a more diverse array of microbes. It also offers a refreshingly crisp bite, thanks to the organic acids that are produced by the millions of microbes that live together in the kefir grains in happy synergy. Like wine, kefir is more of an acquired taste, so don't be surprised if it takes a few tries before you're hooked.

1 tablespoon kefir grains
1⅔ cups (400 ml) whole milk
½ cup extra-ripe berries, or fruit of choice (optional; for the second ferment)

Equipment
One 24-ounce (or 750 ml) glass jar with lid, sterilized
Wooden spoon
Sieve
Funnel
One 24-ounce (or 750 ml) glass bottle or jar, for finished kefir

1. Place the kefir grains in the jar, then pour in the milk. Stir with the wooden spoon and tighten the lid (if you like a fizzy kefir) or loosely cover with the lid (if you prefer a flatter kefir). Leave at room temperature (ideally, 68 to 77°F/20 to 25°C) for 8 hours, out of direct sunlight. Periodically, shake the jar to circulate the grains.

2. Stir the kefir and taste the milk (not the grains). If the milk is still a little watery, leave for an additional 4 to 8 hours. Again, periodically shake the jar to circulate the grains. If you prefer a more sour-tasting milk or live in a cooler climate, you may wish to leave your ferment for up to 48 hours, but if you've tightened the lid, be sure to release the gas by lifting the lid every 8 hours or so.

3. Once it's reached your desired taste and consistency, pour the kefir and grains through the sieve. Using the funnel, transfer the kefir milk to the airtight glass bottle and either store in the fridge, ready for use, or begin the optional second ferment. Depending on how often you drink the kefir, you can repeat the process by adding the strained grains into a fresh jar of milk, or store the grains (see storage tips on page 303).

4. For the optional second ferment: Add the berries to the bottle of kefir. Stir and tighten the lid (if you like a fizzy kefir) or loosely cover with the lid (if you prefer a flatter kefir).

5. How long you let your kefir ferment is up to you. Taste the kefir at least every 8 hours to get a feel for how the flavor changes over time (and, importantly, to let the built-up gas out). The second ferment can take anywhere from 8 to 48 hours, depending on the fermenting conditions.

6. Once you're happy with the taste, chill in the fridge, then serve.

In the first fermentation, lactose, or milk sugar, is the microbe's food, and milk fat helps to protect the microbes during the transit through the acidic environment in the stomach. In the second fermentation, the microbes feed on the fructose, or fruit sugar, from the berries.

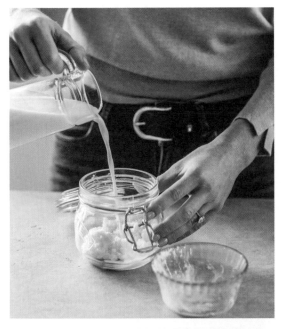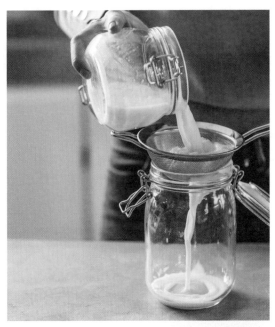

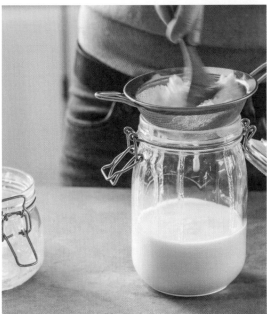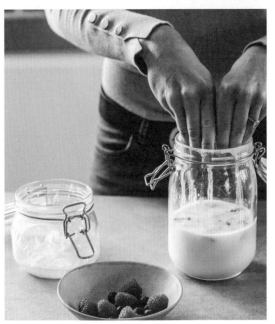

Fermentation produces a range of organic acids that give the kefir a pleasantly sour smell—this is completely normal. For those new to fermenting who may be a little hesitant, your senses will be quick to tell you if something's gone bad—trust me. If you need a reminder of the difference, go and smell some milk that has gone bad.

Water Kefir

If you're looking for a dairy-free drink, water kefir has you covered. Although not directly related to dairy kefir, the grains look similar (but they're more translucent, as in the photo opposite). Dairy kefir survives on lactose (milk sugar), whereas water kefir thrives on sucrose (table sugar).

2 cups (500 ml) warm filtered water

2 teaspoons fresh lemon juice

2 tablespoons sugar (granulated, brown, and natural cane sugar all work and will create slightly different flavors)

2 tablespoons water kefir grains

1 dried fig, free of sulfur-containing additives or oils (see Note)

Second ferment
2½ tablespoons (25 g) ripe berries or fruit of choice, chopped

Equipment
One 24-ounce (or 750 ml) glass jar with lid, sterilized
Wooden spoon
Sieve
Funnel
One 24-ounce (or 750ml) pitcher
One 24-ounce (or 750 ml) airtight glass bottle or jar, for finished kefir

1. Pour the water and lemon juice into a glass jar, add the sugar, and stir with a wooden spoon to dissolve. Once the water has cooled, add the kefir grains and fig, then loosely cover with the lid. Leave at room temperature (ideally, 68 to 77°F/20 to 25°C) for 8 to 12 hours, out of direct sunlight. Periodically, shake the jar to circulate the grains.

2. Stir the kefir and taste the water (not the grains). If the water is still completely flat and sweet, leave for an additional 4 to 8 hours. Warning: Water kefir grains are much more active than milk kefir, so, if you do tighten the lid, be sure to release the pressure by loosening it every 4 to 8 hours, depending on your climate.

3. Once you can taste a slight fizz, pour the kefir and grains through a sieve, catching the kefir water in the pitcher. Discard the fig, then, using the funnel, transfer the kefir water to the airtight glass bottle. Depending on your kefir demand, you can repeat the process by adding the strained kefir grains to a fresh jar of sugar water, or store the grains (see Storage Tips).

4. For the optional second ferment, add the fruit to the bottle of kefir water. Seal the lid to trap in the carbon dioxide, which will give it a refreshing fizz.

5. How long you let your kefir ferment is up to you. Taste your kefir at least every 4 to 8 hours to get a feel for how the flavor changes over time. If you forget to let the gas out every 4 to 8 hours, before doing so, place it in the fridge to cool down and open it away from your face outside, just to be on the safe side (treat it like a champagne bottle—water kefir really can give off a big pop!). The second ferment can take anywhere from 4 to 24 hours, depending on the fermenting conditions and your taste preferences (the longer you leave it, the more acidic the bite).

6. Once you are happy with the taste, chill in the fridge, then serve.

> NOTE: *The fig adds a touch of nutrition for extra healthy microbes. Best to add in every third batch to avoid overfeeding.*

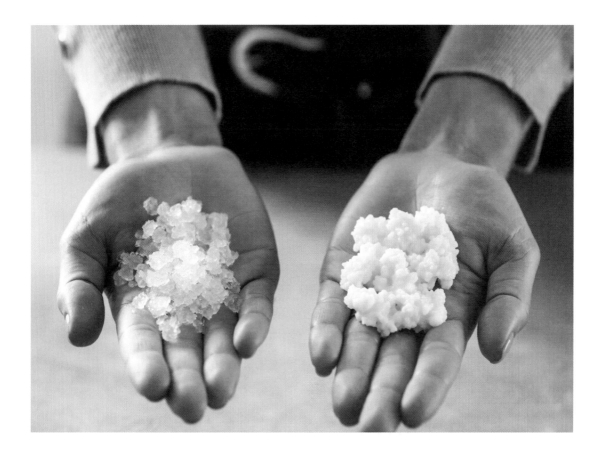

Frequent consumer (at least 1⅔ cups/400 ml a week): This is me. When my first batch of kefir is ready, I strain my grains and add them to a fresh pitcher of milk/sugary water, repeating steps 1 and 2. Once it has reached a few hours shy of my desired taste, I pop the whole jar in the fridge, where I keep it until I've gone through my first batch of kefir. While it's in the fridge, the fermentation continues, but at a much slower rate (dairy kefir keeps in the fridge for up to a week; water kefir two weeks). I then remove it from the fridge and follow step 3.

Infrequent consumer (or if you're going on vacation): You have a couple options. 1) Give it to a friend to "kefir sit": Add the grains to the milk/sugar and store in the fridge with the lid sealed tight. Once every two weeks, your sitter will need to change the milk/sugary water. 2) Freeze: Pat the kefir grains dry, then place in an airtight container/ziplock bag. When you return, place the frozen grains in milk/sugary water to defrost and start at step 1. It will take a few batches before your kefir is back to its bubbly self.

Your kefir grains will double in size every few weeks. As the proportion of grains to milk/water increases, it will ferment faster and faster. It's best to keep the grain:milk/water ratio at around 5 percent and 8 percent, respectively, to prevent over-fermenting. Why not gift your excess grains to friends and family?

Sprouting Seeds and Legumes

This is a staple in my Gut-Goodness Bowls (page 246). Don't feel you should be limiting them to one dish, though; the nutty flavors and crispy crunch make for the perfect high-protein topper in any meal.

¼ cup alfalfa sprouting seeds, dried peas, or dried chickpeas (see Note)
¾ cup (180 ml) filtered or dechlorinated water

Equipment
Sieve
One 24-ounce (or 600 ml) wide-mouth glass jar, sterilized
Cheesecloth (to cover)
Rubber band

1. Day 1: Using the sieve, rinse the seeds well. Place them in the jar and cover with the water (the seeds/legumes will increase a lot in size, so resist the temptation to add extra seeds into the jar). Cover with the cheesecloth and secure with a rubber band. Leave to soak overnight at room temperature (ideally, 65 to 75°F/18 to 24°C).

2. Day 2: In the morning, using the sieve, drain, rinse, and drain again. Cover again with the cloth. Invert the jar and rest it at an angle, using the side of a bowl to hold the bottom of the jar up. This will allow the air to circulate and excess water to drain off. In the evening, repeat the rinsing and draining—this is important to prevent mold from growing on your sprouts (in warm climates, you may need to repeat the rinsing and draining process up to four times a day).

3. Days 3 to 8: Repeat step 2, until 90 percent of the seed jackets have fallen off, in the case of alfalfa, or once the tails are as long as the legume itself.

4. Day 9: Rinse and drain one last time. For alfalfa, pat dry, place in the airtight sterilized jar, and store in the fridge until ready to eat. For legumes, transfer to a saucepan of water and bring to a boil; reduce the heat and boil gently for 45 minutes (for a more firm legume to add to salads) or 60 minutes (for a softer legume perfect for hummus; see recipe on page 264); let cool, pat dry, and store in the airtight sterilized jar in the fridge, ready to use.

NOTE: *To be extra safe, it's best to buy seeds and legumes specifically for home sprouting; they're available from most plant shops.*

Broccoli sprouts are one of the best sources of a phytochemical called glucosinolate. Glucosinolates are converted (with help from your GM) into the almighty antioxidant sulforaphane. This phytochemical is linked with a decreased risk of cancer and heart disease.

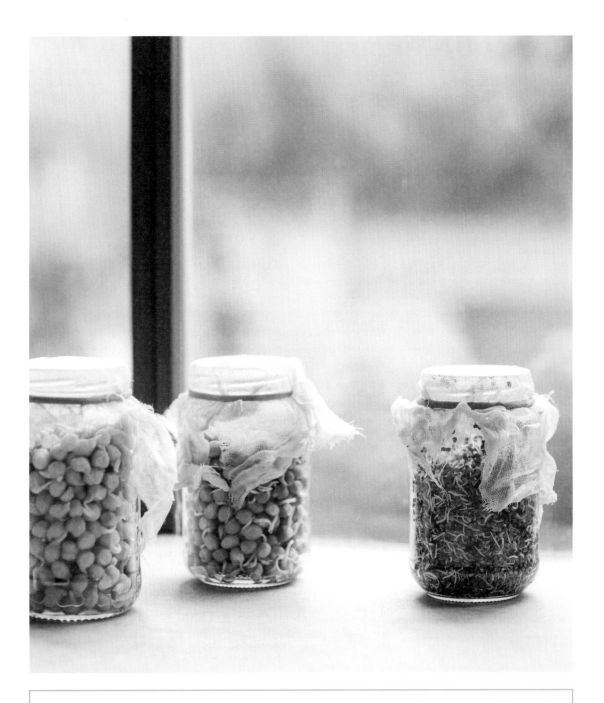

STORAGE TIP: *Alfalfa sprouts will last in the fridge for 1 to 2 weeks. Cooked legumes will keep in the fridge for around 4 days.*

Probiotic Yogurt

Not only does yogurt make a great snack on its own, but its creamy consistency has also earned it a place in many of my recipes, including sauces, dips, and baking. The benefits of yogurt extend beyond the live microbes. Alongside the lactic acid, it also provides 25 percent of most people's daily calcium needs.

Yogurt
2½ cups (600 ml) whole milk (whole milk makes a thicker, creamier yogurt)
1 tablespoon milk powder (optional; for an extra-thick yogurt)
2 tablespoons live plain yogurt (check the label for a yogurt that contains "live cultures" or "probiotics")

Blueberry Chia Jam (optional)
1 cup (140 g) blueberries (or berry of choice)
1 Medjool date, chopped
1 tablespoon chia seeds

Equipment
One 24-ounce (or 750 ml) ovenproof jar, sterilized
Thermometer

1. To make the yogurt, place the milk and milk powder, if using, in a saucepan over medium-low heat and gently simmer until it reaches around 115°F (45°C).

2. Put the live yogurt (the source of the microbes) in an ovenproof jar and slowly stir in the warmed milk so that the yogurt is evenly dispersed.

3. To create the warm environment that makes the yogurt microbes flourish—their preferred temperature is around 105 to 115°F (40 to 45°C), there are several methods (including yogurt makers, which I prefer), but the oven works just fine. Heat the oven to 150°F (65°C), then turn it off. Turn on the oven light, then place the open jar in the oven. The light will keep the oven at a consistent temperature of around 105 to 115°F (40 to 45°C). Leave the jar in the oven for 8 to 12 hours. The longer the incubation period, the thicker and tarter the yogurt.

4. Carefully remove the jar of yogurt from the oven. Allow it to cool on the kitchen counter before placing it in the fridge to set.

5. To make the blueberry chia jam, put the blueberries in a small saucepan, then add the date and ½ cup (120 ml) water. Bring to a gentle simmer (but don't boil). Using the back of a spatula, squish the blueberries and date, then simmer for 10 minutes.

6. Stir in the chia seeds and continue to simmer until the mixture starts to thicken (2 to 3 minutes). Remove from the heat and let cool.

7. To serve, stir in a scoop of the jam with each serving of yogurt.

> STORAGE TIP: *The yogurt keeps in the fridge for up to a week. The chia jam keeps in the fridge for up to 2 weeks.*

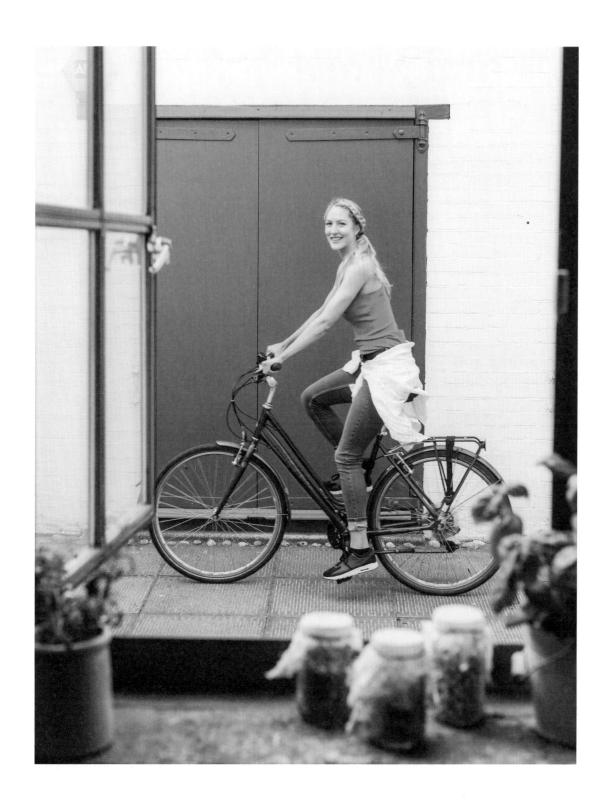

A Final Word

Now you've got everything you need to get started on your gut-health journey. I've personally seen this journey genuinely transform the lives of my patients, and it's not just my own experience talking—it's a powerful concept backed by a wealth of science, which continues to expand. Taking control of their gut health has helped people regain their confidence; improve their quality of life; revive their love of food; defy the odds; prevent family history of chronic diseases, such as diabetes; manage other conditions, including heart disease; and so much more. Gut health is truly revolutionizing our approach to health and wellness, and embracing this vast, untapped resource that lives within each and every one of us is a game-changer.

I hope this book continues to inspire you throughout your journey. No matter how slow or how small your steps, I promise you, it will be worth it. This area is not just my job—it's my passion—and for a long time I've wanted to put all the knowledge and real-world clinical experience I've gained, alongside the landmark research being done around the world, into one place that's easily accessible for all. I hope I've given you a framework with which you can build your own unique gut-health journey and feel empowered to improve your health and happiness. I know you have so much potential to take this knowledge and continue on your journey, and I'm confident you will see results. So, with that, I will leave it in your capable hands.

Notes

Part One: Your Gut Health Guide

1. Svedlund, J. et al., "GSRS—a Clinical Rating Scale for Gastrointestinal Symptoms in Patients with Irritable Bowel Syndrome and Peptic Ulcer Disease," *Digestive Diseases and Sciences* 33 (February 1988): 129–34.

2. Lewis, S. J. et al., "Stool Form Scale as a Useful Guide to Intestinal Transit Time," *Scandinavian Journal of Gastroenterology* 32, no. 9 (September 1997): 920–24.

3. Kort, R. et al., "Shaping the Oral Microbiota Through Intimate Kissing," *Microbiome* 2, no. 1 (November 2014): 41.

4. Reeves, M. et al., "Fat and Fibre Behaviour Questionnaire: Reliability, Relative Validity and Responsiveness to Change in Australian Adults with Type 2 Diabetes and/or Hypertension," *Nutrition & Dietetics* 72, no. 4 (December 2015): 368–76.

5. Jacka, F. et al., "A Randomised Controlled Trial of Dietary Improvement for Adults with Major Depression (the 'SMILES' Trial)," *BMC Medicine* 15, no. 23 (January 2017).

6. Hills, P. et al., "The Oxford Happiness Questionnaire: A Compact Scale for the Measurement of Psychological Well-Being," *Personality and Individual Difference* 33, no. 7 (November 2002): 1073–82.

7. Maier, L. et al., "Extensive Impact of Non-Antibiotic Drugs on Human Gut Bacteria," *Nature* 555, no. 7698 (March 2018): 623–28.

8. Takada, M. et al., "Beneficial Effects of *Lactobacillus casei* Strain Shirota on Academic Stress-Induced Sleep Disturbance in Healthy Adults: A Double-Blind, Randomised, Placebo-Controlled Trial," *Beneficial Microbes* 8, no. 2 (2017): 153–62.

9. Thaiss, C. et al., "Persistent Microbiome Alterations Modulate the Rate of Post-Dieting Weight Regain," *Nature* 540 (November 2016): 544–51.

10. Rossi, M., "Nutrition: An Old Science in a New Microbial Light," *Journal of Human Nutrition and Dietetics* 32, no. 6 (December 2019): 689–92.

11. Gill, S. et al., "Dietary Fibre in Gastrointestinal Health and Disease," *Nature Reviews Gastroenterology and Hepatology* (March 2020).

12. Cade, J. et al., "Dietary Fibre and Risk of Breast Cancer in the UK Women's Cohort Study," *International Journal of Epidemiology* 36, no. 2 (January 2007): 431–38.

13. Tang, G. et al., "Meta-Analysis of the Association Between Whole Grain Intake and Coronary Heart Disease Risk," *The American Journal of Cardiology* 115, no. 5 (December 2014): 625–29.

14. Reynolds, A. et al., "Carbohydrate Quality and Human Health: A Series of Systematic Reviews and Meta-Analyses," *Lancet* 393, no. 10170 (February 2019): 434–45.

15. FoodData Central, U.S. Department of Agriculture, fdc.nal.usda.gov.

16. Sood, A. et al., "The Probiotic Preparation, VSL#3 Induces Remission in Patients with Mild-to-Moderately Active Ulcerative Colitis," *Clinical Gastroenterology and Hepatology* 7, no. 11 (November 2009): 1202–09.

17. Najjar, A. et al., "The Acute Impact of Ingestion of Breads of Varying Composition on Blood Glucose, Insulin and Incretins Following First and Second Meals," *British Journal of Nutrition* 101, no. 3 (June 2008): 391–98.

18. Mozaffarian, D et al., "Changes in Diet and Lifestyle and Long-Term Weight Gain in Women and Men," *New England Journal of Medicine* 364, no. 25 (June 2011): 2392–2404.

19. Dimidi, E et al., "Fermented Foods: Definitions and Characteristics, Impact on the Gut Microbiota and Effects on Gastrointestinal Health and Disease," *Nutrients* 11, no. 8 (August 2019): 1806.

20. "Identification of the 100 Richest Dietary Sources of Polyphenols," *European Journal of Clinical Nutrition* 64, no. S3: S112–20.

21. Clune, S. et al., "Systematic Review of Greenhouse Gas Emissions for Different Fresh Food Categories," *Journal of Cleaner Production* 140 (January 2017): 766–83.

22. Rossi, M. et al., "Dietary Protein-Fiber Ratio Associates with Circulating Levels Of Indoxyl Sulfate and P-Cresyl Sulfate in Chronic Kidney Disease Patients," *Nutrition, Metabolism & Cardiovascular Diseases* 25, no. 9 (September 2015): 860–65.

23. Bokulich, N. et al., "A Bitter Aftertaste: Unintended Effects of Artificial Sweeteners on the Gut Microbiome," *Cell Metabolism* 20, no. 5 (November 2014): 701–03.

24. Suez, J. et al., "Artificial Sweeteners Induce Glucose Intolerance by Altering the Gut Microbiota," *Nature* 514 (September 2014): 181–86.

25. Ibid.

26. Chen, L. et al., "Modest Sodium Reduction Increases Circulating Short-Chain Fatty Acids in Untreated Hypertensives: A Randomized, Double-Blind, Placebo-Controlled Trial," *Hypertension* 76, no. 1 (June 2020): 73–79.

27. Almario, V. et al., "Burden of Gastrointestinal Symptoms in the United States: Results of a Nationally Representative Survey of Over 71,000 Americans," *The American Journal of Gastroenterology* 113, no. 11 (November 2018): 1701–10.

28. Labus, J. S. et al., "The Visceral Sensitivity Index: Development and Validation of a Gastrointestinal Symptom-Specific Anxiety Scale," *Alimentary Pharmacology & Therapeutics* 20 (2004): 89–97.

29. Bessa, O., "Tight Pants Syndrome: A New Title for an Old Problem and Often Encountered Medical Problem," *Archives of Internal Medicine* 153, no. 11 (June 1993): 1396.

30. Okhuysen, P. et al., "Post-Diarrhea Chronic Intestinal Symptoms and Irritable Bowel Syndrome in North American Travelers to Mexico," *The American Journal of Gastroenterology* 99, no. 9 (September 2004): 1774–78.

31. Yao, C. K. et al., "Review article: insights into colonic protein fermentation, its modulation and potential health implications," *Alimentary Pharmacology & Therapeutics* 43, no. 2 (January 2016): 181–96.

32. GBD 2017 Gastro-Oesophageal Reflux Disease Collaborators, "The Global, Regional, and National Burden of Gastro-Oesophageal Reflux Disease in 195 Countries and Territories, 1990–2017: A Systematic Analysis for the Global Burden of Disease Study 2017," *Lancet Gastroenterology and Hepatology* 5, no. 6 (June 2020): 561–81.

33. Lomer, M. C. E. et al., "Review Article: Lactose Intolerance in Clinical Practice—Myths and Realities," *Alimentary Pharmacology & Therapeutics* 27, no. 2 (January 2008): 93–103.

34. Milan, A. et al., "Comparison of the impact of bovine milk β-casein variants on digestive comfort in females self-reporting dairy intolerance: a randomized controlled trial," *The American Journal of Clinical Nutrition* 111, no. 1 (January 2020): 149–60.

35. Skodje, G. et al., "Fructan, Rather Than Gluten, Induces Symptoms in Patients With Self-Reported Non-Celiac Gluten Sensitivity," *Gastroenterology* 154, no. 3 (February 2018): 529–39.

36. Ruxton, C. H. S., "The Impact of Caffeine on Mood, Cognitive Function, Performance and Hydration: A Review of Benefits and Risks," *Nutrition Bulletin* 33, no. 1 (March 2008): 15–25.

Heckman, M. et al., "Caffeine (1, 3, 7-trimethylxanthine) in Foods: A Comprehensive Review on Consumption, Functionality, Safety, and Regulatory Matters," *Journal of Food Science* 75, no. 3 (2010): R77–R87

37. Zong, G. et al. "Abstract 11: Associations of Gluten Intake with Type 2 Diabetes Risk and Weight Gain in Three Large Prospective Cohort Studies of US Men and Women," *Circulation* 135, suppl. 1 (March 2018): A11.

38. Carr, S. et al., "CSACI Position statement on the testing of food-specific IgG," *Allergy, Asthma & Clinical Immunology* 8, no. 1 (July 2012): 12.

39. Roe, M. et al., "*McCane and Widdowson's The Composition of Foods* Seventh Summary Edition and updated Composition of Foods Integrated Dataset," *Nutrition Bulletin* 40, no. 1 (March 2015): 36–39.

40. Lovell, R. et al., "Global prevalence of and risk factors for irritable bowel syndrome: a meta-analysis," *Clinical Gastroenterology and Hepatology* 10, no. 7 (March 2012): 712–21.

41. Drossman, D. et al., "International Survey of Patients With IBS: Symptom Features and Their Severity, Health Status, Treatments, and Risk Taking to Achieve Clinical Benefit," *Journal of Clinical Gastroenterology* 43, no. 6 (July 2009): 541–50.

42. Chumpitazi, B. P. et al., "Review article: the physiological effects and safety of peppermint oil and its efficacy in irritable bowel syndrome and other functional disorders," *Alimentary Pharmacology and Therapeutics* 47, no. 6 (March 2018): 738–52.

43. Khanna, R. et al., "Peppermint oil for the treatment of irritable bowel syndrome: a systematic review and meta-analysis," *Journal of Clinical Gastroenterology* 48, no. 6 (July 2014): 505–12.

44. Furnari, M. et al., "Clinical trial: the combination of rifaximin with partially hydrolysed guar gum is more effective than rifaximin alone in eradicating small intestinal bacterial overgrowth," *Alimentary Pharmacology & Therapeutics* 32, no. 8 (October 2010): 1000–06.

45. Khalighi, A. R. et al., "Evaluating the efficacy of probiotic on treatment in patients with small intestinal bacterial overgrowth (SIBO) - A pilot study," *Indian Journal of Medical Research* 140, no. 5 (November 2014): 604–08.

46. Tuck, C. J. et al., "Increasing Symptoms in Irritable Bowel Symptoms With Ingestion of Galacto-Oligosaccharides Are Mitigated by α-Galactosidase Treatment," *American Journal of Gastroenterology* 113, no. 1 (January 2018): 124–34.

47. Vanuytsel, T. et al., "Psychological stress and corticotropin-releasing hormone increase intestinal permeability in humans by a mast cell-dependent mechanism," *Gut* 63, no. 8 (August 2014): 1293–99.

48. Al Khatib, H. K. et al., "The effects of partial sleep deprivation on energy balance: a systematic review and meta-analysis," *European Journal of Clinical Nutrition* 71, no. 5 (May 2017): 614–24.

49. Watson, N. F. et al., "Transcriptional Signatures of Sleep Duration Discordance in Monozygotic Twins," *Sleep* 40, no. 1 (January 2017): zsw019.

50. Liu, Y. et al., "Prevalence of Healthy Sleep Duration among Adults—United States, 2014," *Morbidity and Mortality Weekly Report* 65, no. 6 (February 2016): 137–41.

51. Reed, P. et al., "Problematic Internet Usage and Immune Function," *PLoS One* 10, no. 8 (August 2015): e0134538.

52. Al Khatib, H. K. et al., "Sleep extension is a feasible lifestyle intervention in free-living adults who are habitually short sleepers: a potential strategy for decreasing intake of free sugars? A randomized controlled pilot study," *The American Journal of Clinical Nutrition* 107, no. 1 (January 2018): 43–53.

53. Lally, P., "How are habits formed: Modelling habit formation in the real world," *European Journal of Social Psychology* 40, no. 6 (October 2010): 998–1009.

54. Zhou, S. et al., "Pharmacological and non-pharmacological treatments for irritable bowel syndrome: Protocol for a systematic review and network meta-analysis," *Medicine* 98, no. 30 (July 2019): e16446.

55. Cohen, S., et al., "A Global Measure of Perceived Stress," *Journal of Health and Social Behavior* 24, no. 4 (December 1983): 386–96.

56. Schumann, D. et al., "Randomised clinical trial: yoga vs a low-FODMAP diet in patients with irritable bowel syndrome," *Alimentary Pharmacology & Therapeutics* 47, no. 2 (January 2018): 203–11.

57. Bennike, I. et al., "Online-based Mindfulness Training Reduces Behavioral Markers of Mind Wandering," *Journal of Cognitive Enhancement* 1 (April 2017): 172–81.

58. Economides, M. et al., "Improvements in Stress, Affect, and Irritability Following Brief Use of a Mindfulness-based Smartphone App: A Randomized Controlled Trial," *Mindfulness* 9, no. 5 (2018): 1584–93.

59. Allen, J. et al., "Exercise alters gut microbiota composition and function in lean and obese humans," *Medicine & Science in Sports & Exercise* 50, no. 4 (April 2018): 747–57.

60. Ibid.

61. Lawrence, J. et al., "Prevalence and co-occurrence of pelvic floor disorders in community-dwelling women," *Obstetrics & Gynecology* 111, no. 3 (March 2008): 678–85.

62. Lämås, K. et al., Effects of abdominal massage in management of constipation—a randomized controlled trial," *International Journal of Nursing Studies* 46, no. 6 (June 2009): 759–67.

Part Two: Recipes

1. Bovier, E. R. et al., "A Double-Blind, Placebo-Controlled Study on the Effects of Lutein and Zeaxanthin on Neural Processing Speed and Efficiency," *PLoS One* 9, no. 9 (September 2014): e108178.

2. Gaforio, J. et al., "Virgin Olive Oil and Health: Summary of the III International Conference on Virgin Olive Oil and Health Consensus Report, JAEN (Spain) 2018," *Nutrients* 11, no. 9 (September 2019): 2039.

3. de Alzaa F. et al., "Evaluation of Chemical and Physical Changes in Different Commercial Oils During Heating," *Acta Scientific Nutritional Health* 2, no. 6 (May 2018): 2–11.

4. Hu, M-L. et al., "Effect of Ginger on Gastric Motility and Symptoms of Functional Dyspepsia," *World Journal of Gastroenterology* 17, no. 1 (January 2011): 105–10.

5. Bonilla Ocampo, D. et al., "Dietary Nitrate from Beetroot Juice for Hypertension: A Systematic Review," *Biomolecules* 8, no. 4 (December 2018): 134.

6. Ried, K., "Garlic Lowers Blood Pressure in Hypertensive Individuals, Regulates Serum Cholesterol, and Stimulates Immunity: An Updated Meta-Analysis and Review," *The Journal of Nutrition* 146, no. 2 (February 2016): 389S–96S.

7. Josling, P., "Preventing the Common Cold with a Garlic Supplement: A Double-Blind, Placebo-Controlled Survey," *Advances in Therapy* 18, no. 4 (July/August 2001): 189–93.

Nantz, M. et al., "Supplementation with Aged Garlic Extract Improves Both NK and γδ-T Cell Function and Reduces the Severity of Cold and Flu Symptoms: A Randomized, Double-Blind, Placebo-Controlled Nutrition Intervention," *Clinical Nutrition* 31, no. 3 (June 2012): 337–44.

8. Schiering, C. et al., "Feedback Control of AHR Signalling Regulates Intestinal Immunity," *Nature* 542 (February 2017): 242–45.

9. Holscher, H. et al., "Walnut Consumption Alters the Gastrointestinal Microbiota, Microbially Derived Secondary Bile Acids, and Health Markers in Healthy Adults: A Randomized Controlled Trial," *The Journal of Nutrition* 148, no. 6 (June 2018): 861–67.

10. Montagna, M. et al., "Chocolate, 'Food of the Gods': History, Science, and Human Health," *International Journal of Environmental Research and Public Health* 16, no. 24 (December 2019): 4960.

11. Grassi, D. et al., "Flavanol-rich chocolate acutely improves arterial function and working memory performance counteracting the effects of sleep deprivation in healthy individuals," *Journal of Hypertension* 34, no. 7 (July 2016): 1298–308.

12. Ried, K., "Effect of Cocoa on Blood Pressure," *Cochrane Database of Systematic Reviews* 2017, no. 4 (April 2017).

13. Hekmat, S. et al., "Survival of *Lactobacillus acidophilus* and *Bifidobacterium bifidum* in Ice Cream for Use as a Probiotic Food," *Journal of Diary Science* 75 (January 1992): 1415–22.

14. Clune, S. et al., "Systematic Review of Greenhouse Gas Emissions for Different Fresh Food Categories," *Journal of Cleaner Production* 140, no. 2 (January 2017): 766–83.

15. Dimidi, E. et al., "Fermented Foods: Definitions and Characteristics, Impact on the Gut Microbiota and Effects on Gastrointestinal Health and Disease," *Nutrients* 11, no. 8 (August 2019): 1806.

16. Fahey, J. W. et al., "Broccoli Sprouts: An Exceptionally Rich Source of Inducers of Enzymes That Protect Against Chemical Carcinogens," *Proceedings of the National Academy of Sciences of the United States of America* 94, no. 19 (September 1997): 10367–72.

17. Aslani, Z. et al., "Lentil Sprouts Effect on Serum Lipids of Overweight and Obese Patients with Type 2 Diabetes," *Health Promotion Perspectives* 5, no. 3 (October 2015): 215–24.

18. He F. et al., "Beneficial effects of potassium," *BMJ* 323 (September 2001): 497–501.

19. Song, H. J. et al., "Consumption of kimchi, a salt fermented vegetable, is not associated with hypertension prevalence," *Journal of Ethnic Foods* 1, no. 1 (December 2014): 8–12.

20. Kontis, V. et al., "Future life expectancy in 35 ndustrialised countries: projections with a Bayesian model ensemble," *Lancet* 389, no. 10076 (April 2017): 1323–35.

Subject Index

Recipe Index

Page numbers in *italics* refer to photos.

Acknowledgments

To my husband, it turns out you're not only a brilliant doctor, but you also have a real flair for editing. Thank you for coming on this journey with me and reading every single word (five times over). Mum, no words can describe how grateful I am for your endless support; without you there would be no book.

To my nutrition and dietetic colleagues who critically reviewed and challenged every page, you have made this book really something special: Dr. Heidi Staudacher, Marianne Williams, Dr. Katrina Campbell, Yvonne McKenzie, Dr. Eirini Dimidi, Dr. CK Yao, Dr. Caroline Tuck, Dr. Samantha Gill, Dr. Ricardo Da Costa, and Dr. Ana Rodriguez-Mateos.

To the microbe experts, Dr. Johan van Hylckama Vlieg, Dr. Erin Shanahan, Professor Julian Marchesi; gut physiologists, Dr. Mark Scott and Dr. Anthony Hobson; gastroenterologists, Professor Douglas Drossman, Dr. Shameer Mehta, Dr. Farooq Rahman, and Professor David Sanders; and immunologist Dr. Jenna Macciochi; thank you for sharing your brains. I have learned so much from all of you.

Niki Webster and Renee Martensen, thank you for your game-changing flavors. To my family, friends, and social media followers for being my recipe testers, and to Claire Hitchen and Jessica Rowan-Parry for reviewing my words—I truly valued every piece of feedback.

To my chapter contributors, Kimberly Wilson, Richie Norton, Dr. Haya Al Khatib, Lucy Allen, and Ellie Bradshaw, your additions have been instrumental in achieving my vision for a holistic guide to the gut.

To Olivia and the team at The Experiment, thank you for believing in my book and helping it change the lives of even more people. To Emily, Richard, Emma, Libby, and the shoot team, what a journey—thank you for going that extra mile. John Hamilton, thank you for sharing your brilliance with me—I am forever grateful. RIP.

And finally, to each and every one of you that has supported The Gut Health Doctor journey. Thank you for believing in my mission—you are my driving force.

About the Author

MEGAN ROSSI, PhD, RD, the Gut Health Doctor, is considered one of the world's most influential gut health specialists. A registered dietitian and nutritionist for the last decade, she has an award-winning PhD in gut health, which was recognized for its contribution to science with the dean's award for outstanding research.

As a leading Research Fellow at King's College London, Megan is currently investigating nutrition-based therapies in gut health, including prebiotics, probiotics, dietary fibers, plant-based diversity, the low-FODMAP diet, and food additives. She established The Gut Health Clinic, where she leads a team of gut-specialist dietitians who are making an evidence-based approach more accessible. More recently, Megan has created her own gut health food company, Bio&Me, to bridge the gap between science and food industry.

Frustrated that her research findings weren't reaching the public, and seeing fad diets and potentially dangerous misinformation on gut health being spread, Megan took to social media to share credible information and science-based advice, building an active community of hundreds of thousands of people.

Aussie-born Megan has also been recognized as *Business Insider*'s Top 100 Coolest People in Food & Drink and was named Young Australian Achiever of the Year.

Love Your Gut is her first book. Originally published as *Eat Yourself Healthy* in the UK, it immediately became an Amazon and *Sunday Times* bestseller.

Connect with Megan at theguthealthdoctor.com

TheGutHealthDoctor

TheGutHealthDoctor

TheGutHealthDoc